Smart Guide™
to
Yoga

About Smart Guides™

Welcome to Smart Guides. Each Smart Guide is created as a written conversation with a learned friend; a skilled and knowledgeable author guides you through the basics of the subject, selecting the most important points and skipping over anything that's not essential. Along the way, you'll also find smart inside tips and strategies that distinguish this from other books on the topic.

Within each chapter you'll find a number of recurring features to help you find your way through the information and put it to work for you. Here are the user-friendly elements you'll encounter and what they mean:

The Keys

Each chapter opens by highlighting in overview style the most important concepts in the pages that follow.

Smart Move

Here's where you will learn opinions and recommendations from experts and professionals in the field.

Street Smarts

This feature presents smart ways in which people have dealt with related issues and shares their secrets for success.

Smart Sources

Each of these sidebars points the way to more and authoritative information on the topic, from organizations, government agencies, corporations, publications, Web sites, and more.

Smart Definition

Terminology and key concepts essential to your mastering the subject matter are clearly explained in this feature.

F.Y.I.

Related facts, statistics, and quick points of interest are noted here.

What Matters, What Doesn't

Part of learning something new involves distinguishing the most relevant information from conventional wisdom or myth. This feature helps focus your attention on what really matters.

The Bottom Line

The conclusion to each chapter, here is where the lessons learned in each section are summarized so you can revisit the most essential information of the text.

One of the main objectives of the *Smart Guide to Yoga* is not only to better prepare you to undertake a yoga practice, but to explain the myriad benefits yoga offers and the many ways that the science can be used to enrich one's life.

Smart Guide™

to

Yoga

Stephanie Levin-Gervasi

Photographs by a. paul cartier

CADER BOOKS

John Wiley & Sons, Inc.

New York • Chichester • Weinheim • Brisbane • Singapore • Toronto

Library of Congress Cataloging-in-Publication Data:
Levin-Gervasi, Stephanie.
Smart guide to Yoga / Stephanie Levin-Gervasi.
p.   cm.
Includes index.
ISBN 0-471-35648-4 (pbk.)
1. Yoga, Hatha. 2. Physical fitness. I. Title.
RA781.7.L478   1999
613.7'.046—dc21   99-31068

Printed in the United States of America

10 9 8 7 6 5 4 3 2 1

*This book is dedicated to
my daughter, Camille,
whose endless inspiration, curiosity, and joy
capture the infinite spirit of the yogi.*

Acknowledgments

I extend my heartfelt gratitude to the yoga teachers and individuals who offered knowledge and insight throughout the book. I especially want to acknowledge Integral Yoga in San Francisco, particularly the Reverend Kamala Lee, whose generosity and clarity have illuminated the heart of yoga for me.

I also would like to thank a. paul cartier, the photographer of the book's interior illustrations. A freelance photographer/imager for more than twenty years, he has sold work to health and travel magazines as well as photographed numerous special events. He is an avid cyclist and yoga practitioner.

Special gratitude also to the models in the photographs, Kriste Home and Joseph Vella. Kriste and Joseph are both certified Integral Yoga instructors. Joseph is a practitioner of Transcendental Meditation as well.

Contents

Introduction

Yoga is a complete science that anyone can practice. This ancient system of integrating physical, mental, and spiritual well-being is the most widely practiced health system throughout the contemporary world. People are drawn to yoga for many reasons, but the most common reason given is to keep the body and mind supple.

The yoga postures in this book exercise the entire body and tone and stretch muscles and joints. The yoga breathing exercises presented will calm and revitalize the mind as well as fine-tune concentration.

Yoga has several branches, and chapter 1 explores these various branches before introducing hatha yoga, the most widely practiced yoga system in the West. The *Smart Guide to Yoga* has as its primary focus the hatha system. This first chapter as well defines yoga and dispels common myths and interpretations that sometimes surround yoga. A very brief history of yoga and the foundation for yoga practice segues into the health benefits yoga offers.

Chapter 2 explores hatha yoga more deeply and delves into the differences and similarities of the various hatha systems one might discover when ferreting out a yoga class.

The next chapter is devoted to pranayama, the life force or energy that is the invisible link to all yoga practices. Pranayama is a science. Simply said, it is the science of breathing correctly. Since stress affects our breath, we conclude this important chapter with some breathing exercises, complete with visuals to aid you in your practice.

A number of hatha yoga poses, or asana, that you will encounter in a hatha class and throughout the book are illustrated with step-by-step instructions in chapter 4. There are asana for beginners, intermediate, and advanced yoga students. Each pose details the translation of the Sanskrit name as well as the primary benefits the pose offers. The chapter concludes with illustrated instructions for the Sun Salutation, the continuous, fluid exercise that stretches and benefits the entire body .

Chapter 5 addresses issues common to finding a class and developing your own yoga practice. It will help you prepare to embark on yoga and offer assistance in finding the right teacher and performing alone at home. There are tips for beginning yoga students and for overcoming common obstacles that can impede a practice.

The differences between the Western and Eastern philosophies in respect to health and the body are used as an introduction to the chapter on chakras. Western thought sees the body and mind as separate entities; Eastern thought sees them as one entity. The energy centers known as chakras—the seven points within our body, each with its corresponding physical function—are essential in Eastern approaches to health and wellness.

Chapter 7 introduces meditation and the various methods people use to meditate. There are helpful hints for the busy mind and some simple practices to focus the mind that can be done at the office or at home, in a backyard or on a plane.

The next two chapters focus on the benefits of yoga specifically to women and to men. Chapter 8 explores yoga and women, including female cycles, pregnancy and prenatal yoga, and perimenopause and menopause. This extensive chapter is full of helpful suggestions and information for adopting yoga and meditation for use through different life passages. The chapter on men and yoga dispels the common "male" myths surrounding yoga and explains the many benefits growing numbers of men reap from the ancient practice.

Yoga's link to health and how yoga has been adopted in the medical and scientific communities are the focus of chapter 10. Here it is explained how yoga is being used to treat such common conditions as coronary heart disease, chronic pain, back pain, stress, arthritis, and carpal tunnel syndrome.

The concluding chapter takes yoga on the road, into the workplace, and right at home for the entire family. Here we have suggestions for incorporating yoga with travel or at the office and with busy schedules; for parents using yoga with their children; and for seniors contemplating a new yoga class or practice. And for those who want to experience yoga in a health club or spa or on a retreat, there are advice and recommendations in the final pages of the book.

Enjoy your journey.

Smart Guide™
to
Yoga

CHAPTER 1

....

Yoga and Its Branches

THE KEYS

• While the word *yoga* has a succinct definition, yoga's meaning—and practice—can be applied in many ways.

• Yes, yoga is shrouded in myths—we dispel them in this chapter.

• Yoga's popularity has grown due to its numerous health benefits. Yoga is a complete tool to keep the body fit and flexible and the mind focused and quiet. It integrates body, mind, and spirit and can be practiced anywhere, by anyone.

• The benefits of yoga are vast and include stress reduction, enhanced mental acuity, increased flexibility, a calm mind, and relief of chronic pain.

• Yoga has its own language—Sanskrit.

• There are six different branches of yoga embracing a multiplicity of styles and techniques and appealing to different personalities.

Yoga, the once serendipitous fad of the 1960s, is at the turn of the century the most widely practiced exercise system in the world. According to *Yoga Journal,* approximately 6 million people practice yoga. Maybe you are one of them, or maybe you have thought about yoga but never found the time to include it in your hectic schedule. On the other hand, perhaps your image of yoga conjures up levitating swamis, venerable vegetarians, and weightless bodies twisting toward infinity. While a few of these descriptions are valid—yes, some yogis do levitate and some physicians urge vegetarian choices—the practice of yoga is as personal as your choice in food or your taste in art.

Yoga is a potent tool for stress reduction, fitness, and mental health. There is a surfeit of yoga schools, teachers, philosophies, and practices, all of which are discussed in this book. Just as we all choose different life routes, and pace ourselves accordingly to reach a personal goal, so this book shows that yoga is a compendium of small routes allowing the individual to travel at his or her own pace. Because yoga has sprouted numerous branches and a diverse assortment of techniques throughout the centuries, the most prudent place to begin your yoga practice is at the beginning, some five thousand years ago.

Yoga Defined

Yoga is a complete exercise system developed more than five thousand years ago in India to energize and strengthen mind-body awareness. A time-honored practice, yoga strives to balance physical health and psychological well-being and to create a sense of inner peace. Devised by ancient sages as a perfect method for self-integration, yoga is today recognized in the West as a potent application for both physical and mental health.

Medical and managed-care facilities around the country are implementing yoga for stress reduction. At Boston's Mind/Body Medical Institute, Dr. Herbert Benson has devised stress-management methods for relaxation that include yoga and meditation. Jon Kabat-Zinn, Ph.D., founder and director of the Stress Reduction Clinic at the University of Massachusetts Medical Center, includes yoga and meditation in his chronic pain clinics. Even a few health maintenance organizations (HMOs) have added yoga classes to their health-education programs.

Yoga has become a staple for many spas and is even beginning to segue into the business sector, with many companies now offering lunchtime yoga classes.

The Practice

The practice of yoga embraces a multiplicity of styles and an astonishing array of diverse techniques, all of which aim to foster holistic harmony. The best way to approach yoga is to find a class. You can read about yoga or watch tapes that can introduce you to yoga, but yoga is like swimming; you have to dive in and do it. You can't experience the crawl, the breaststroke, or synchronized breathing until you get wet. The pleasure of floating on your back in a warm pool cannot be experienced in a book or a photograph; you have to submerge your body. To experience the effects of

SMART DEFINITION

Yoga

A Sanskrit word derived from the word *yuj*, literally meaning "yoke together" or "union." The underlying purpose of yoga was to unite the individual self with the Divine.

The correct pronunciation is *YO-gah*.

Yogi

Pronounced *YO-gee*, a man who practices yoga.

Yogini

Pronounced *YO-gee-nee*, a woman who practices yoga.

SMART SOURCES

The Yoga Research
   Society
341 Fitzwater St.
Philadelphia, PA 19147
(215) 592-YOGA

The Yoga Research
Society holds a yearly
conference that brings
together authors,
researchers, doctors,
and others to share
knowledgeable
perspectives on yoga.

yoga, you have to breathe, stretch, and focus on quieting your active mind.

Dispelling Common Myths about Yoga

Myth: You have to be deeply religious to practice yoga.
Fact: Anyone can practice yoga. You do not have to be religious, nor is there any imposing prerequisite or lifestyle that you must adhere to. Because yoga does not have its roots in a Western tradition, some people find the spiritual component of yoga oddly exotic. If you already have a spiritual inclination or practice, yoga will enrich it.

Myth: You have to be flexible and already in good shape to practice yoga.
Fact: You do not have to be svelte or have the body of Madonna and the flexibility of a gymnast to reap the benefits that yoga has offered millions all over the world.

Myth: People who do yoga are vegetarians who go along with New Age philosophies and trends.
Fact: You do not have to be a vegetarian, swear off caffeine, or wear beads to try yoga. Yoga is "ageless"—it is for everyone, of every age group—and it is not a New Age invention or a religion.

Myth: People who practice yoga do it so they can become "enlightened."
Fact: Yoga is not a spiritual light bulb that lights up when you have a problem or need to chill out. It

does, however, encourage people to self-introspection. There may be a subtle shift in your attitudes and habits after practicing yoga for a while. You might decide to start the day with a quiet walk or find it easy to stop smoking. You may feel the desire to change your diet or moderate your eating habits.

Why Is Yoga Suddenly So Popular?

While the wisdom of yoga blossomed in India centuries ago, the interest in yoga in the West is just beginning to bloom.

Why the interest in yoga all of a sudden? That depends on the perspective of the person practicing yoga. Some speculate that we are more open to the esoteric and medicinal influences of yoga and are more willing to embrace traditions from other cultures. The landslide of yoga classes in universities and health centers speaks to a generation with a profound interest in physical and mental health.

The baby boomers, some of whom practiced yoga as an exercise in the counterculture of the '60s, continue to show an unquenchable interest in the therapeutic effects of yoga. Still others discover yoga out of desperation. They are in pain and disenchanted with traditional medical modalities for backaches, headaches, and general malaise when they turn to yoga as an alternative.

In a yoga class of a dozen people, everyone may have a different reason for being in the class. Because human beings reflect a vast range of emotional, mental, and physical capacities, people approach yoga for many different reasons.

SMART SOURCES

Looking for a yoga class at your YMCA? Call YMCA of the U.S.A.'s toll-free number for more information:

(800) USA-YMCA
[800-872-9622]

A Brief History of Yoga

The phenomenon of yoga has inspired a scholarly, spiritual, and personal interest in some of yoga's ancient writings and language. There are magazines on yoga, and hundreds of articles about yoga are published yearly. But from where does all this interest stem, and how did it come about?

Yoga's Scholarly Contribution

The earliest reference to yoga is in the Vedas, India's oldest texts on religion and mysticism, written between 2500 B.C. and 600 B.C. Scholars consider the Vedas the sacred seeds that later flourished into India's religious and philosophical practices.

The Vedic people inhabited the Indus Valley from around 1800 B.C. to 1000 B.C. The concept of altering one's consciousness appears to have played a rather dominant role in Vedic society.

Much later, an isolated group of self-seekers began a more mystical search for transcendentalism. They became known as Upanishads and authored writings on the means of achieving enlightenment. *Upanishads* is a Sanskrit word that means "to sit next to." Before the phenomenon of yoga classes, yoga was taught one on one, handed down orally from teacher to student. Both the writings in the Vedas and Upanishads texts were concerned with the spiritual component of yoga. It was the *Bhagavad Gita,* a national cherished Hindu epic text that contains essential yoga concepts, that first espoused other yoga practices.

Yoga's Contemporary Contribution

In 1928 Paramahansa Yogananda, a spiritual master, left India and came to California. He was not the first yogi to come to America and practice yoga, but he was one of the first Indian masters to live in the West. He practiced kriya yoga, a technique that consists of body discipline, mental control, and meditating with an emphasis on pranayama (a component of yoga defined later in this chapter). His book, *Autobiography of a Yogi*, first published in 1946, introduced thousands of Americans to the concepts and practice of yoga. He founded the Self-Realization Fellowship in California, a yoga center that has flourished and still practices and teaches pranayama techniques.

In 1934 Yogananda predicted that there would come a time when the message of yoga would sweep the world.

Yogananda's message came to fruition thirty years later.

In the late 1960s, Americans and Europeans, seeking extraordinary experiences, went to India. Yogis who had never been out of India ventured across the ocean and came to America and Europe to teach yoga. Like Yogananda, some established yoga centers. By the late '60s, anything that came from India was labeled yoga, and yoga became a nonconventional mix of teaching that embraced spirituality, health, and an alternative lifestyle.

However, the conventional American was still not interested in swamis and alternative forms of relaxation. The ancient Indian science, shrouded in the mists of time, and practiced for centuries in rural villages without electricity or water, eventually reached millions of mainstream Americans by way of television. It was not a bearded Indian sage Americans tuned into, but a health-conscious man by the name of Richard Hittleman.

Richard Hittleman

Richard Hittleman offered the public a single, simple exercise plan that required a minimum of effort to attain maximum results.

In 1961 Hittleman took his exercise plan to the airwaves, and his nationally syndicated yoga show aired from Los Angeles. It was an instant success and remained on television for many years.

Hittleman authored some of the first books on yoga—*Yoga for Health* and *Yoga 28-Day Exercise Plan.*

Lilias Folan

Not long after Hittleman's successful program on yoga, a housewife by the name of Lilias Folan launched her PBS series *Lilias, Yoga & You,* in 1970. Her popularity soared, and yoga gained an even wider audience.

Folan authored *Lilias, Yoga and Your Life.* Both Richard Hittleman's and Lilias Folan's enthusiasm for yoga encouraged millions of people to investigate and practice yoga.

By the late 1970s and early 1980s yoga was inching its way into universities, churches, and community centers. Hundreds of yoga centers and ashrams, most of them practicing something called hatha yoga, sprouted across America.

Since that time yoga has mushroomed. Countless yoga centers, community centers, YMCAs, and fitness facilities now teach yoga.

F.Y.I.

Stress is linked to hypertension, heart attacks, diabetes, asthma, chronic pain, allergies, headaches, backaches, and immune system weakness.

Seventy-five to 90 percent of employee visits to hospitals are for ailments linked to stress.

Sources: American Institute of Stress; *Nation's Business,* December 1994; respectively.

F.Y.I.

Coronary Heart Disease (CHD) is the single largest killer of American males and females. In 1995, coronary heart disease caused 481,287 deaths in the United States.

Source: American Heart Association

Some individuals regard yoga as a practical adjunct to their life—they feel better. Others practice yoga for physical, psychological, or spiritual reasons—their body feels more flexible, they sleep better, or they become more aware of their beliefs.

The Benefits of Yoga

Ancient yoga masters considered good health to be an integrated state of physical, mental, and social well-being. Because it is a profound tool to restore balance to the whole person, yoga affords many benefits in areas such as:

- **Cardio, respiratory, and circulatory health.**

- **Stress reduction.** Reducing stress is one of the paramount health concerns in people's lives today.

- **Mental relaxation.** In order to completely relax the body, one must first learn to relax the mind.

- **Pain relief.**

- **Flexibility and toning.** There is no other exercise that tones and maintains flexibility as well as yoga does.

- **Body position and movement awareness.**

- **Interdependent functioning of the mind and body.** Yoga is an exacting exercise that engages both the body and mind.

Yoga and Heart Health

Cardiologist Dr. Dean Ornish was one of the early pioneers to incorporate yoga into his medical research. In the early 1970s, Ornish was a young medical student in Texas, specializing in cardiology. During medical school Ornish was introduced to yoga through his family. He understood the positive effects yoga had on his life, and he began doing research.

He approached a number of cardiologists about referring coronary heart patients to his research study called "The Effect of Yoga and a Vegetarian Diet on Coronary Heart Disease." The overall response went something like this: "I'd like to support your research, but it sounds too weird. What would I tell my patients, that I'm referring them to a swami?"

The idea that heart disease is reversible and that heart patients might fold into a pretzel on a floor bordered on medical heresy. Eventually, Dr. Ornish changed the name of his study to "Effects of Stress Management Techniques and Dietary Changes on Coronary Heart Disease" and got his patients as well as a little funding.

The Language of Yoga

The original language and text of yoga is Sanskrit. Nevertheless, yoga has been translated into untold numbers of other languages for use by the cultures of the world. But whether you take yoga classes in India, Iowa, or Ireland, Sanskrit is the language used to identify everything from the yoga poses (asana) to the breathing exercises (pranayama).

Understandably, until your ear warms up to the linguistic flow of Sanskrit, it can sound like Urdu. Not to worry, though. Sanskrit as translated phonetically into English is an easy language, pronounced precisely as it is written. And the images in yoga translate smoothly into vivid English.

F.Y.I.

The *Bhagavad Gita*, which is contained in the national epic *Mahabharata*, is perhaps the best known of all yogic scriptures. It is an epic conversation between the incarnated god Krishna and the warrior-prince Arjuna. As Prince Arjuna prepares for battle, he realizes that his cherished teacher and friend will be his opponent. Lord Krishna instructs Prince Arjuna on the correct ways to live fully and meaningfully in the world. It embodies both spiritual and mundane struggles and how to act accordingly in full consciousness of the divine.

Sanskrit 101

Before starting yoga, you'll need to acquaint yourself with some some simple Sanskrit words commonly used in classes (and this book).

Asana

Asana refers to the physical component of yoga. Practicing asana requires an awareness of your body, your posture, and gravity. The spine is of particular importance in asana because it is the central supporting system for your entire body. If your day has ever been foiled by a back attack, you understand how intimately the spine is connected to other body parts. All asana, whether they are done sitting, standing erect, or standing on your head, involve movement of the spinal column.

Pranayama

Pranayama refers to breath control or the breathing exercises in yoga. *Prana* is the vital force or life energy, and *yama* means "to extend." In yoga it is the awareness of the breath that helps move you fluidly through the asana. Some forms of yoga concentrate solely on the breath, and without incorporating the breath, you're not actually doing yoga. Pranayama is also the catalyst for relaxation and may be practiced alone or with the postures.

Pratyahara

Pratyahara refers to sensory detachment. It is a discipline to control the senses and the mind. Pratyahara quiets the senses, drawing them away from stimuli in order to meditate. Our senses are natural conduits for stimulation—not all bad, of course. Nevertheless, one cannot hope to meditate if the senses are engageded. In yoga, in order to attain an actual state of meditation, one must learn to withdraw from the senses. This is done through breathing exercises, which ultimately help to quiet the mind in preparation for meditation.

Who Is a Guru?

A guru is a sage of steady wisdom, a teacher who shows you the way. As the distinguished Indian yoga master T. K. V. Desikachar wrote in his classic *The Heart of Yoga*: "A guru is not one who has a following, a guru is one who encourages and shows the way."

India does not have a patent on gurus. Other traditions, like the martial arts, also have knowledgeable masters to teach or show the way. In India, it is the guru who traditionally imparts the spiritual knowledge of yoga to his student. In Japan, the *sensei,* similar to the guru, is the mentor who instructs his students in the physical and mental components of the martial art.

Gurus are spiritual mentors, not molds to be cloned. They are gifted human indicators, rich in wisdom, knowledge, and clarity. A true guru directs you and helps you find your own path or your own voice. Some people search out gurus, and others haven't the slightest interest in ever meeting one. When choosing a yoga class you may encounter teachers or yoga centers that follow a specific yoga lineage or philosophy based on the teachings of a guru. This doesn't mean that you have to follow that particular spiritual philosophy to practice yoga. You may never come in contact with the teachings of a guru, and you do not need a guru to practice yoga.

In Praise of Patanjali and the Eight Limbs

If you practice yoga for a good amount of time, Patanjali's name will crop up. Patanjali was a sage and a physician who lived somewhere between 200 B.C. and 200 A.D. No one knows the exact date of his birth or death. Patanjali codified his knowledge and thoughts on yoga, which became *The Yoga Sutras of Patanjali*. Pantanjali extracted the parts of the Vedas that dealt with mastering the mind, updated the language, and modernized these verses. The 195 sutras are aphorisms or precise parables to reflect on and incorporate into your life. Sutras define the entire science of yoga, and for this reason Patanjali is often called the "Father of Yoga." The sutras, although translated, are best understood by discussion in a class.

Patanjali's writings have been described as "the epitome of tolerance." *The Yoga Sutras of Patanjali* is considered the most fundamental text on the system of yoga, covering everything from social responsibility to how to concentrate the mind. The heart of his teachings are the eight limbs or the eightfold path of yoga, known as ashtanga yoga.

The Eight Limbs

These eight limbs, known as angas, are a progressive series of disciplines; they are not, however, prerequisites to practice yoga. Great—so why mention them?

Because the eight limbs are yoga's ethical blueprint, the moral codes of a vast tradition. Many who practice yoga want to know more about the philosophy and spiritual content contained within these interdependent guidelines which focus on ethics, attitudes, and interactions.

The eight limbs are prescriptives to cultivate body, mind, and spiritual awareness and to examine habitual attitudes, behaviors, and reactions—if you choose to do so. The limbs are not linear, but intertwine, much the way branches do in a forest. They require discipline and concentration. If you thrive on instant gratification, some of the limbs that require dedication will seem as foreign as cold soup for breakfast. On the other hand, if you consider yourself a relatively moral being, you may already practice some of the limbs; they are universal.

Yama

This limb examines social behavior and is the foundation for all the other practices. The five yamas are nonviolence; truth and honesty; nonstealing and forbearance; moderation; and nonpossessiveness.

Niyama

The limb examines inner discipline and responsibility. The five niyamas are purity; contentment; austerity; study of the sacred text; and living with an awareness of the Divine.

Asana

This limb is solely concerned with maintaining steadiness and control of the body. Asana prepares the body for meditation. Ancient yogis realized that in order to sit and contemplate, the body needed to be supple and cooperative.

Pranayama

The vehicle for meditation, pranayama is the breath, and it helps maintain equilibrium in the body.

Note: Asana and pranayama will be part of any hatha yoga class. The following four limbs evolve sequentially and require practice.

Pratyahara

This limb deals with withdrawing the senses in order to still the mind. Pratyahara happens during meditation, when the senses are not stimulated.

Dharana

This limb strives to fix the mind on one point or image. When this happens, the mood is set for the seventh limb.

Dhyana

This is uninterrupted meditation without an object. Inner dialogue disappears and the mind is keenly focused.

Samadhi

This is when all the limbs work. There are no impediments to block your path.

The Branches of Yoga

The elegance of yoga is that the more you learn, the deeper the experience and the more beneficial. There are, however, different kinds of yoga that appeal to a range of individuals.

Some people have to experience yoga physically; they find meditating or relaxing too challenging. Others have a deep urge to understand and intellectualize their yoga practice, and the physical component of yoga may not take priority. There are those who cannot imagine yoga without a relationship with the Divine—people who practice the yoga of devotion, meditation, service, knowledge, and study—and there are many who never incorporate religious beliefs into their yoga practice at all. Some people chant, others are more contemplative.

If this is your initial foray into yoga, investigate the different practices and methods and pick the one that works best for you. No matter what type of yoga or combination of yoga styles you choose to practice, the effects of your practice will be cumulative on your body, mind, and lifestyle. Yoga is not a static practice; it encourages you to investigate various techniques and teachers.

The most widely practiced yoga tradition in the West is hatha yoga (which is physical yoga; this is the branch of yoga that this book will primarily focus on). However, there are five other branches or paths of yoga as well. Many people practice just one branch of yoga, while others integrate a few together. Just as we all have different learning preferences—some of us are somatic, others of us are visual or auditory—we may feel more comfortable with one branch of yoga rather than another, because of the way we assimilate information or learn. The six branches of yoga to explore are the following:

- **Raja,** yoga of physical and mental control

- **Karma,** yoga of action

- **Jnana,** yoga of knowledge or wisdom

- **Bhakti,** yoga of love and devotion

- **Tantra,** ritual yoga to awaken energy in the body

- **Hatha,** physical yoga

Raja Yoga

The classical, nonphysical yoga system used for meditation is called raja yoga. *Raja* means "king" and raja yoga is known as the royal path. Raja yoga requires a fair amount of study or knowledge of the yoga traditions and the sutras. This form of yoga is primarily intended for those who prefer to gain insight through practical or empirical experience. The eight limbs of yoga are studied and are incorporated into one's lifestyle. In raja yoga the individual practices certain mental exercises and meditation under the tutelage of a teacher or guru. The aim of these exercises and study is to attempt to observe the true light or the individual's true inner nature. Raja yoga leads the individual to direct personal experiences of deeper levels into his or her own being. When the mind is clear, the royal power within each of us can surface. When the mind is not restless, this is raja yoga.

SMART SOURCES

The Shri Ram Chandra Mission is one source for information about books, seminars, member services, and research on raja yoga.

http://www.srcm.org/ index.html

SMART SOURCES

The SpiritWeb site offers a series of eleven lessons in karma yoga, including a history and a detailed outline of the process of thought and practice of karma. Also available is a link to a calendar of events.

http://www.spiritweb. org/Spirit/Yoga/ karma-yoga.html

Karma Yoga

Karma is the yoga of action, and it focuses on the causes and effects of an individual's actions. The goal of karma yoga is to guide one to spiritual freedom through selfless service to others. Karma achieves union with God through right action and through service. Individuals practicing karma yoga do not receive rewards for good deeds, nor is karma yoga attached to a specific outcome. The individual performs a service without judgment, expectation of a desired outcome, or a reward for the action. Those who practice karma yoga are not vested in a positive or negative result. Since actions are not performed for self-gratification, the person performing the service is completely involved in what he or she is doing. Focus is totally in the moment without worry of success, failure, or ego. The ego is sublimated in karma yoga.

Jnana Yoga

Jnana yoga is the search for knowledge and wisdom and is considered a somewhat difficult path. Before embarking on the jnana path, one must integrate the wisdom of the other branches of yoga into his or her life. It serves individuals with strong intellectual interests and those whose philosophical ideas and search for truth are of critical importance in determining the direction of their lives. The awareness in jnana is always inward, and the jnana yogi uses his or her mind to inquire into his or her own nature. Jnana assumes all knowledge is within us, although it is not always apparent. It is up to the individual to uncover this dormant knowledge. The

SMART SOURCES

For more information on jnana yoga, including books, courses, lectures, and conferences, check out the following site:

http://www.hatem.com/ jnana.htm

jnana yogi embarks on a three–step process: he or she listens to, reflects on, and recognizes knowledge, and then tries to integrate these three components of knowledge together. Jnana is philosophical; it is a perfect type of yoga for the individual who desires to move past material reality. Jnana yogis find knowledge through God.

Bhakti Yoga

Bhakti yoga is the mystical path of personal devotion, and it relates well to emotional expression. Its aim is to open the heart by selfless love and devotion. The heart is bhakti yoga's focus. Through the heart, bhakti achieves unity with the Divine. The term *bhakti* means "to serve the Divine." In bhakti a union with the Divine occurs through prayer, worship, and ritual. It is achieved by love alone, love not of a person but of a higher power. Bhakti places devotion to the Divine above all intellectual or material concerns in the world. The bhakti yogini acts out of conviction and is completely devoted to God. Enlightenment for a bhakti yogini is through selfless love and devotion to the Divine.

Tantra Yoga

Tantra yoga is probably the most misunderstood yoga system in the West. It is often misquoted as a means to sensual indulgence. It is not a yoga of isolation or for ascetics. Tantra yoga uses all the natural senses and desires with the aim to transform and harmonize these senses and desires. Tantra yoga works with the highly charged energy in the

SMART SOURCES

For a comprehensive guide to bhakti yoga with notes by Sri Swami Sivananda, check out the following site on the Internet:

http://blizzard.rsl.ukans.
edu/~pkanagar/divine/
teachings/bhaktiyoga.
htm

SMART SOURCES

An introduction to tantra yoga can be found at the Abhidhyan Yoga Institute web site. This page offers advice, recommended readings, and information on training sessions and lectures.

http://www.abhidhyan.
org

body called kundalini. The kundalini sits coiled at the base of the spine and is often blocked. Kundalini can be uncoiled only by guided proper breathing techniques. Mystical yet scientific in approach, tantra yoga includes visualization, chanting, asana, and strong breathing practices. For the tantric yogi, the Divine can be found in ordinary, day-to-day existence. Tantra embraces the physical world rather than a world of withdrawal.

Tantra yoga should always be guided or taught by a teacher due to the overpowering effect of the kundalini awakening spontaneously.

Hatha Yoga

Hatha yoga aims to strengthen and tone the body as well as free the mind from distraction. Hatha represents the duality in life—yin and yang, masculine and feminine, darkness and light. The Sanskrit word is made up of *ha,* which represents the sun, and *tha,* which represents the moon. Hatha yoga joins these dual forces; it is the yoga of physical well-being, designed to balance the body's opposing forces. Hatha was originally intended to stabilize and relax the body in preparation for long periods of sitting meditation. Perhaps hatha has been so popular in the West because it is concrete and less spiritual. One can actually see and feel the body in asana and see its progress.

While hatha yoga styles vary greatly, all hatha yoga has evolved from one origin or discipline. How the asana are done and where the attention is focused may change dramatically between teachers and styles. Some hatha schools emphasize mastering the form of the posture, while others are not as concerned with the structural outcome of a posture as they are with deriving a sense of fluidity and inner peace when doing the postures. A few schools of yoga crank up the heat to rid the body of impurities, and other schools use props for the asana. There are yoga teachers that give a modicum of instruction, while others are more detailed. There are schools with flexible approaches that integrate several different hatha approaches to yoga, and other less lenient schools that adhere to one distinct approach.

You will have to find the approach that best suits your personality. No matter what the approach, keep in mind that the asana have been tempered in many instances to reflect on our Western body types and lifestyles.

Okay, maybe you're thinking, Boy, this is a far cry from putting on a leotard or a pair of baggy pants and a shirt, throwing a towel on the floor, and physically rolling into postures. Or perhaps you're thrilled—you're not the physical type and you are glad to know that there are other avenues or paths to yoga, that there is much more to yoga than just physical postures. As you have seen, there are six distinct branches of yoga practice that you might encounter on your search for a yoga class.

However, the most common type of yoga practiced is hatha yoga, and the majority of people interested in yoga seek out hatha. So it is wise to look at the different schools of hatha before beginning a class. The next chapter explores the numerous choices and diversity within the hatha yoga system and gives an introduction to the essential asana (posture work) and pranayama (breathing exercises).

THE BOTTOM LINE

Yoga strives to balance the mind, body, and inner peace. Anyone can do yoga, and people choose to practice yoga for diverse reasons. The top three reasons people practice yoga are to reduce stress, to become more anatomically flexible, and to relax the mind. The phenomenon of yoga has inspired a scholarly, spiritual, and personal interest in some of yoga's ancient writings and language. While yoga is not a religion, it incorporates the teachings and philosophies of world religions. Some people find following the spiritual teachings of a guru the best approach to yoga; others are just as happy to take a yoga class once a week. Most yoga practitioners do hatha, or physical, yoga—which is just one of the six diverse branches of the practice.

The Different Systems of Hatha Yoga

In response to an endemic interest in fitness and health, yoga's popularity has soared, giving rise to a number of yoga schools. Sleuthing through the library of lineages can be intimidating for a beginning yoga student. Classes, instructors, and techniques vary; what does not vary is yoga's goals: to calm the mind and to cultivate a state of alert relaxation.

The most popular of the yoga schools is hatha yoga. This chapter introduces different styles of hatha yoga and teachers who brought hatha yoga to the West. Also introduced is the asana, the physical or tangible principle of yoga that is widely practiced in the West.

Hatha Yoga

Approximately 85 percent of the people who practice yoga practice hatha, or physical, yoga. Hatha yoga has become synonymous with bending, stretching, twisting, and standing on your head. This is a bit of a distorted picture of hatha. Hatha yoga uses a series of slow, gentle movements strung together by breathing and concentration. Through a series of poses or postures, breathing techniques, and concentration hatha yoga works to weave the breath, body, and mind together.

A movement or posture can be something as simple as standing erect and consciously raising your arms to the sides of your body, or it can be something a little more complicated, such as lying on the floor on your stomach, bending your knees, and reaching back with both hands to grab your ankles and put the body into a bow position.

Though the systems of hatha yoga vary—there

are enough Westernized versions of this ancient Indian discipline to make even the most liberal yogi leery—the benefits are unmatched: balance, strength, flexibility, and a reprieve from life's unrelenting static.

Some hatha approaches you will encounter refer to a particular teacher who has refined his method, while others refer to a particular yoga practice. Some of the approaches are rigorous or more physically demanding, while others have a definite meditative or therapeutic quality about them.

These hatha yoga approaches were brought to the West by yoga masters, many of whom were either strongly influenced by or studied with a man by the name of Sri Krishnamacharya.

Sri Krishnamacharya

Krishnamacharya was born in India in 1888 into a family that practiced yoga. He later went to Banaras and learned yoga from some of India's best teachers and then to Bengal to study Ayurvedic medicine, the Indian system of healing. As an Ayurvedic doctor, he used yoga in his practice, prescribing yoga on an individual basis. He is considered the foremost source regarding yoga theory and application, and he practiced yoga until his death in 1989. He is credited with developing four different branches of yoga in his lifetime and teaching some of the great yoga teachers. Several of Krishnamacharya's students incorporated his teachings into their methods and carried them to the West.

SMART DEFINITION

Ayurvedic medicine

A medical science that originated in India five thousand years ago. Ayurveda is based on the existence of a primal energy. Ayurveda postulates that when an individual's energy flow is smooth, health is maintained. Ayurveda recognizes the importance of mind-body balance.

STREET SMARTS

Annie McQuid managed a yoga studio in Portland, Oregon, where she taught different styles of yoga. When she moved to San Francisco to manage and teach at Shala Yoga, someone suggested she take an ashtanga yoga class. "I had been teaching prenatal yoga, which is pretty low key. I wasn't sure I would resonate with ashtanga; now I've incorporated it into my teaching."

SMART SOURCES

For more information about ananda yoga contact:

The Expanding Light Retreat
14618 Tyler Foote Road
Nevada City, CA 95959
(800) 346-5350

Hatha Yoga Systems

In your search for the "right" yoga class, you may shop around and try a few different venues. The first thing you'll notice is that one teacher has a precise way of teaching a pose while another teacher changes the pose slightly. Sometimes teachers may even refer to the same pose by a different name. Or you may hear someone say, "I'm doing kripalu," or "I'm into kundalini," and wonder if these are actually yoga classes. They are. In fact, hatha yoga is no longer the generic yoga of the 1960s but over the last few decades has evolved into several different approaches.

The following is a brief list of the hatha yoga schools with a description of their focus, followed by a more in-depth explanation of the methods and the founding practitioners.

- **Ananda**, strong emphasis on meditation

- **Ashtanga**, strong emphasis on the physical

- **Bikram**, emphasis on the physical and sweating

- **Integral**, emphasis on relaxation by integrating positions, breath, and meditation

- **Iyengar**, emphasis on symmetry and alignment

- **Kripalu**, emphasis on flowing and merging of body, breath, and mind

- **Kundalini**, focus is on the breath

- **Sivananda**, emphasis is on integrating positions, breath, and meditation, and is gentle

• **Viniyoga**, emphasis is on integrating poses and breathing for the individual, and breathing is stressed

Ananda

Ananda yoga was developed by an American named Donald J. Walters, known as Swami Kriyananda. He founded the Ananda Ashram, located at the Ananda community in Nevada City, California.

Ananda yoga is linked to the yoga of Paramahansa Yogananda's teachings. Swami Kriyananda devoted forty-five years of his life to disseminating Yogananda's teachings. Ananda yoga uses asana to clear and energize the body in preparation for meditation while simultaneously focusing on the postures to heighten self-awareness. The use of affirmations is a distinct feature of ananda yoga. In class, the emphasis is placed on deeply relaxing and focusing on the asana. Ananda yoga is gentle in its approach.

Ashtanga

K. Pattabhi Jois, a Krishnamacharya disciple, is credited with developing the physically challenging style of hatha yoga known as ashtanga, which is not to be confused with the eightfold path of ashtanga. Ashtanga is the power of yoga, and some refer to it as "power yoga."

Ashtanga yoga is an active yoga practice sometimes compared to the intensity of an athletic workout. In ashtanga yoga, a sequence of set poses, beginning with what is known as the Sun Saluta-

SMART DEFINITION

Ashram

A physical setting where a community of people practice a certain type of yoga. Some ashrams are small; others resemble small cities. A core of people who practice yoga live and run the ashram. Yoga classes, workshops, and teachers' training are offered at ashrams across America.

SMART SOURCES

For more information on power yoga, check out the following site:

www.poweryoga.com

The New York Road Runners Club offers information on classes, descriptions, and how to learn more about power yoga.

www.nyrrc.org/powyog. htm

tion, are repeated in a continual flow, which links the movements and the breath. This intense flow creates heat that produces a cleansing or detoxifying effect associated with this method. It is not unusual to see students wipe their brow with a towel or drink water during a ninety-minute class. Class ends with relaxation techniques. Generally, ashtanga students tend to be fit and on the younger, athletic side, although there are older individuals who practice ashtanga. K. Pattabhi Jois's institute is in Mysore, India.

Bikram

Bikram Choudhury created a technique using an exact set of twenty-six postures, which focus on cleansing the body from the inside out. Two pranayama (breathing) techniques are included in a class, one at the beginning and one at the end. This style of yoga has been called the "yoga to the stars" because several famous people in Hollywood have studied Bikram.

This practice is rigorous and not easy; it's a *workout*. During a class, the postures are repeated twice and held for at least ten seconds. You must be fit for this routine, and if you have injuries, this may not be the yoga method for you. For even more of a challenge during class, the thermometer is turned up to around 85 degrees and the room is very hot and steamy. Plan to sweat here.

Bikram schools are called the Yoga College of India. There are schools in Tokyo, Honolulu, San Francisco, and Beverly Hills. Bikram Choudhury has been at the center in Beverly Hills since the 1970s. The Beverly Hills Yoga College of India is where the teacher's training program takes place.

Integral

The integral yoga system was developed by Swami Satchidananda, the author of the book *Integral Hatha Yoga* and numerous other texts on yoga. Swami Satchidananda introduced yoga to America at Woodstock, when he led thousands in chanting "Om" for peace. He was Dr. Dean Ornish's teacher, and many of Swami Satchidananda's therapeutic aspects of yoga are used in medical settings around the country. He has synthesized many different types of yoga and stresses a life lived simply, peacefully, and usefully. A sense of well-being and peace dominates the ninety-minute yoga classes, which follow a set format, including forty-five minutes of positions, deep relaxation, and meditation. Emphasis is placed on relaxation, alignment, and finding your comfort center while practicing yoga.

Swami Satchidananda established the Integral Yoga Institute in 1966, and it now has more than forty branches worldwide. The main headquarters is at Satchidananda Ashram–Yogaville, in Virginia. Besides offering courses in raja yoga and yoga classes specifically designed for people with injuries or physical problems, the institute offers an in-depth, teachers' certificate training program.

Iyengar

The Iyengar approach to yoga may be the most widely practiced form of yoga in the West. As a teenager in Pune, B. K. S. Iyengar suffered from malaria, typhoid fever, and respiratory difficulties. Stricken by poverty and disease for much of his young life, Iyengar was neither flexible nor strong

SMART SOURCES

For more information on integral yoga, contact:

Satchidananda
   Ashram–Yogaville
Buckingham, VA 23921
(804) 969-3121
(800) 858-YOGA

Integral Yoga Institute
770 Dolores St.
San Francisco, CA
   94110
(415) 824-9600

For more information on Iyengar yoga, contact:

Iyengar Yoga Institute
   of San Francisco
2404 Twenty-seventh
   Avenue
San Francisco, CA
   94116
(415) 753-0909

STREET SMARTS

Rona Edmunds began practicing yoga thirty years ago. "I didn't feel whole in my life and knew I needed to make a change. I was living near the kripalu center and decided to take the teachers' training." Rona says kripalu is based on the psychologist Carl Rogers's philosophy. In kripalu, once an individual understands what is happening emotionally and physically in his or her body and mind, he or she has the choice to modify it.

SMART SOURCES

For more information on kripalu, contact:

Kripalu Center
Box 793
Lenox, MA 01240
(800) 967-3577

as a young man. He was discouraged from studying yoga and began to teach himself the practice. Mastering his own frail health, he began teaching others and studied with Krishnamacharya.

Iyengar has a rigorous and scientific approach to hatha yoga. He stresses understanding the body and how it works. His emphasis is on alignment and props for individual needs. Iyengar introduced props—such as chairs, ropes, sandbags, and blankets to aid in yoga—and these props have become a benchmark of his technique.

The focus in an Iyengar class is on symmetry. There may be a lot of standing poses in beginning classes. Because postures require a change of props, the flow of a class can vary greatly. Iyengar has an intense, long, and rigorous teachers' training program.

Iyengar's school, Ramamani Iyengar Memorial Yoga Institute, named after his wife, is in Pune, India, and attracts people from all over the world to study with Iyengar.

Kripalu

Kripalu yoga is an internal-directed approach developed by Yogi Amrit Desai. Desai was influenced by an Indian master who practiced kundalini (the freeing of energy) and focused on pranayama (breathing techniques). Desai came from India in the 1960s to study at a design school in Pennsylvania. He taught yoga to make extra money.

Kripalu yoga has three stages. The first stage is the actual, steady practice of the postures and their basic mechanics. Good body alignment is coordinated with breathing and movement. In this stage, one works with his or her own strength and weakness in the postures. The postures are generally held for a short period of time.

During the second stage, the postures are held longer and the teacher addresses the students' mental and emotional states while doing the postures. In this stage a teacher will encourage the student to feel what is going on in the body both emotionally and physically. For example, the mind might be concentrated on a feeling of not really wanting to do the posture or on a thought such as "I might break my neck if I try this posture."

The third stage of kripalu surrenders to the body's own wisdom. As in Desai's own experience, this means actually doing postures spontaneously. Desai calls this "meditation in motion."

The atmosphere in kripalu is noncompetitive, and it is also taught one-on-one. Kripalu offers a strong teaching certification program at their headquarters in Lenox, Massachusetts. For the moment, there are no other kripalu centers in the country, although there are teachers elsewhere who teach kripalu.

Kundalini

Sikh Yogi Bhajan, Ph.D, brought kundalini yoga to the West in 1969. For thousands of years this practice has been carefully handed down from master to disciple by oral tradition. Kundalini yoga has always been somewhat of an obscure, guarded secret in India. It was never taught publicly until Yogi Bhajan challenged tradition and began teaching kundalini yoga in the West.

Kundalini is the ancient practice designed to awaken the kundalini, or coiled energy, stored at the base of the spine. In yoga, the kundalini en-

SMART SOURCES

For more information regarding kundalini yoga contact:

3HO International
  Headquarters
P.O. Box 351149
Los Angeles, CA
  90035
(310) 552-3416

STREET SMARTS

Nidhi Adhiya grew up in India where she practiced hatha yoga as a child. While modeling and acting in New York, someone suggested she try kundalini yoga. "I loved the energy and calmness it gave me; I'd never experienced anything like it before. It altered my life direction. I'm now a yoga teacher, and I commute between Los Angeles and New York teaching kundalini."

SMART SOURCES

For more information on sivananda yoga contact:

Sivananda Yoga
  Vendanta Center
1200 Arguello Blvd.
San Francisco, CA
  94122
(415) 681-2731

Sivananda Yoga
  Vendanta Center
243 West 24th Street
New York, NY. 10011
(212) 255-4560

ergy is represented by a coiled snake. The prana (another word for vital force or energy) cannot flow until the snake begins to uncoil. Unfortunately, this area of the body holds much tension and blocks the path of prana.

Kundalini mixes chanting, breathing practices, and yoga exercises that involve the physical body, the auric body, and magnetic fields to move this energy up the spine. The emphasis is not on asana but rather on chanting and breathing. Chanting is done in large groups with a partner. The chanting creates an invigorating and calming experience. Kundalini's primary focus is the power of the breath. Kundalini has been defined as an evolutionary force within us.

Yogi Bhajan encourages followers to focus on an integrated lifestyle of health and well-being, practicing everything from a good diet to community service. Yogi Bhajan's Healthy, Happy, Holy Organization is headquartered in Los Angeles and New Mexico. There are fifteen hundred kundalini teachers worldwide. Kundalini should always be taught with a teacher who practices and understands kundalini. This is not a hatha yoga style to learn on your own.

Sivananda

The sivananda style of yoga was founded by Swami Vishnu Devananda, a promoter of traditional hatha yoga. He studied various styles of yoga for ten years before he came to the West. In 1958 he authored a very thorough guide to yoga called *The Complete Illustrated Book of Yoga,* which was published in 1960. It set the tone for many of the first yoga classes taught in this country.

During a ninety-minute class, sivananda yoga incorporates proper asana, breathing, and deep relaxation. Sivananda yoga works with the basic principles of asana, meditation, and deep relaxation. A vegetarian diet and positive thinking with meditation are encouraged for a healthy lifestyle.

Sivananda yoga classes are gentle in approach and usually follow the twelve postures found in the Sun Salutation. Classes are easy to follow and begin with short chants and conclude with deep relaxation and a closing chant. The environment is relaxed and gentle. There are six sivananda centers located in North America and India.

Viniyoga

T. K. V. Desikachar is Krishnamacharya's son. He teaches yoga and carries on the traditions of his father at the school named in honor of his father, Krishnamacharya Yoga Mandiram, in Madras, India. Desikachar has pioneered medical research with yoga on conditions such as schizophrenia, depression, asthma, and diabetes. His style of hatha yoga is an individualized, step-by-step approach called viniyoga. The emphasis in viniyoga is twofold. It recognizes the uniqueness of the individual and creates an approach using all the tools of yoga, including asana, chanting, pranayama, and meditation, and it teaches the yoga practitioner how to apply these tools in individual practice. The approach is relaxed and the pace is gentle. Viniyoga's strength is that it modifies postures to the needs of the individual student. A profound awareness of the breath is central in viniyoga, and inhalation and exhalation are stressed a great deal throughout a class. The asana become an expression of the

SMART SOURCES

Many yoga teachers incorporate components of viniyoga into their classes. The following are sources specifically for viniyoga.

Gary Kraftsow
1030 E. Kuiaha R.
Haiku, Maui, HI 96708
(808) 572-1414

New Dawn Yoga
  Therapy
Dawn Summers
P.O. Box 460395
San Francisco, CA
  94146-0395
(415) 285-1831

Julie Rappaport
(415) 263-3940
San Francisco, CA
julesr@slip.net
www.slip.net/~julesr/

www.heartofyoga.org

Margaret and Martin
  Pierce
Pierce Program
1164 N. Highland Ave.
  N.E.
Atlanta, GA 30306
(404) 875-7110

breath. If the breath is strong and flowing, so is the body. There is less stress on the joints and knees in viniyoga compared to some other types of hatha yoga because the postures are done with slightly bent knees. An overall sense of well-being predominates in viniyoga classes. Viniyoga is beginning to be used in therapeutic environments.

Emerging Styles of Yoga

Yoga was carried to this country by yoga mavericks or masters who founded their own distinct styles of hatha yoga and were both adept and persistent in their teachings. Within America, there have also been Americans who have discovered new approaches and styles of teaching yoga.

Restorative Yoga

Restorative yoga is a gentle style of yoga that uses props to facilitate relaxation as well as help support the body in the asana. Isn't all yoga restorative? Yes, yoga is designed to help the individual feel integrated or whole as well as relaxed. And in most traditional hatha yoga classes, the sessions begin with active poses, such as the Sun Salutation or forward-bending poses. The classes typically wind down with restful or restorative poses. In restorative yoga, however, all the poses or asana are restorative in nature.

How Restorative Yoga Works

Judith Lasater, Ph.D., P.T., author of *Relax & Renew: Restful Yoga for Stressful Times* and often called the "mother of restorative yoga," refers to restorative yoga as "active relaxation."

By supporting the body with blankets, bolsters, or pillows, the poses stimulate and relax the body as it strives toward balance. Some of the poses in restorative yoga benefit the entire body; others benefit individual areas; all reduce the effects of stress. Restorative yoga works all the spinal muscles and stimulates and soothes internal organs.

The best time to practice is when you feel fatigued or tired. Restorative yoga helps to rebalance the body during menstruation or menopause and during times of emotional stress.

Finding a Restorative Yoga Class

The best way to learn restorative yoga is to take a class. Your teacher will show you how to use the props effectively and how to improvise with props at home. Many yoga teachers are beginning to incorporate restorative poses into their classes.

Phoenix Rising

Developed by Michael Lee in 1984, Phoenix Rising Yoga is based on the kripalu method, and it is a combination of classical yoga poses married to elements of mind-body psychology. It's immensely therapeutic, incorporating poses for inner awareness, mental acuity, emotional stability, and physical balance, as well as spiritual awareness.

Phoenix Rising has sixteen basic poses and is

SMART SOURCES

Phoenix Rising Yoga
   Therapy
P.O. Box 819
Housatonic, MA 01236
(800) 288-9642

For a directory of Phoenix Rising yoga teachers around the country, go to the web site:
http://www.yogasite.
   com/teachers.html

SMART SOURCES

Kali Ray Tri-Yoga Center
113 New Street and
   708 Washington
   Street
Santa Cruz, CA
(831) 464-8100
Mailing address:
P.O. Box 4287
Santa Cruz, CA 95063

Kali Ray Tri-Yoga Center
Route 7, Sheffield, MA
(413) 229-3399
Mailing address:
P.O. Box 321
Great Barrington, MA
   01230

done with a therapist who gently holds the student until emotional tension surfaces and is released. Through assisted yoga postures, guided breathing, and nondirective dialogue, Phoenix Rising aims to connect the physical and emotional halves of the self. A one-on-one discussion follows with a guided meditation.

Tri-Yoga

This flowing, dancelike approach to hatha yoga was founded by Kali Ray, who is also the director of the tri-yoga center in Santa Cruz, California. Tri-yoga incorporates a series of continuous, precise flowing postures and integrates asana, pranayama, and meditation. The mood is meditative.

The practice has seven levels, ranging from basic beginning to advanced. Tri-yoga consists of a spontaneous, dance-related series of poses accompanied by background music. Each series or level of poses prepares you for the next level. In all levels, tri-yoga works with the body's flexibility, strength, endurance, and the mind's knowledge of the tri method. The sequences in class are repeated, deepened, and elaborated upon. The careful incremental approach emphasizes breath, mudra (hand postures), and energy flow. Tri-yoga is considered therapeutic. Classes conclude with a seated pranayama and meditation.

Power Yoga

Power Yoga™, founded by Beryl Bender Birch and Thom Birch, is based on ashtanga yoga (see page

25). This physical form of yoga incorporates both a strong mind and body workout. Practiced in a sequence of postures, power yoga builds strength and focus while unwinding tight joints and muscles.

The Asana

The backbone of hatha yoga are the poses, or postures, and these are called asana. The asana are fluid movements that stretch the muscles and tone the body and are held from several seconds to a few minutes. If you aren't flexible or if you're used to moving slowly, you may feel intimidated or uncomfortable with how the body moves. This will pass. The body in yoga is like an instrument: when you first practice, it may seem out of tune, but the more you practice yoga, the more in tune you become with your body.

We'll focus more on the asana, and illustrate the most common poses, in chapter 4.

Pranayama

Asana requires good breathing skills; it is the breath that helps you maximize each asana. Pranayama is the science of breathing; how you breathe is as important as the pose.

You'll be encouraged to think about how you breathe and then to concentrate on your inhalation (inward breath) and your exhalation (outward breath). You might find inhaling easier than exhaling or vice versa. The key to breathing in yoga is to first become aware of how you breathe.

THE BOTTOM LINE

Hatha yoga is no longer generic but encompasses a variety of techniques. The philosophy of yoga remains the same but the teaching methods differ. Sri Krishnamacharya was one of the greatest teachers of the century, inspiring many teachers who brought their own techniques to the West.

There is a yoga style for every personality. Investigate the different styles of yoga before choosing a class. Viniyoga is a gentle, individual approach, as are kripalu, integral, and sivananada. Ananda's gentle approach also incorporates the use of affirmations. Kundalini yoga does not focus on asana but uses breathing, chanting, and other techniques to access the body's energy. Ashtanga, Bikram, and Iyengar are considered more strenuous. Remember: yoga is personal, and though styles vary, the benefits are the same.

Pranayama: The Science of Breathing

Breathing is a continuous, exact process, yet we pay scarce attention to our breath. Breath is life. Our lungs are the bridgeway to our oxygen supply. It is the automatic act of breathing that carries oxygen to the blood and brain and controls the flow of prana, our vital energy.

"It is as difficult to explain prana as it is to explain God," wrote B. K. S. Iyengar in *Light on Pranayama: The Yogic Art of Breathing.* "Prana is the energy permeating the universe at all levels. It is physical, mental, intellectual, sexual, spiritual, and cosmic energy. All vibrating energies are prana. It is the hidden or potential energy in all beings, released to the fullest extent in times of danger. It is the prime mover of all activity. It is energy which creates, protects, and destroys. Vigor, power, vitality, life, and spirit are all forms of prana."

Let's begin to scratch the surface.

Pranayama

Pranayama is made up of two words: *prana,* which is "life force" or "energy," and *yama,* which is "discipline." Pranayama is the discipline of breathing, a vast science of breath control. The objective of pranayama is to increase physical and mental health. In advanced pranayama practices, there are various ways to achieve this.

Entire books have been written on pranayama. In yoga, prana is the powerful life force and it exists in everything, both positive and negative. Prana is much more than breathing in oxygen and expelling carbon dioxide; it is the backbone of a good yoga practice.

Western science cannot verify the existence of this subtle energy force. Nevertheless, this energy is very much a part of Eastern medicine. For example, acupuncture balances the flow of the body's energy, known as chi, through a system of meridians.

In yoga, this subtle energy is prana. In addition to the physical body, yogis believe that the individual has an astral body or an emotional body. Prana is the life energy that is the link between the physical and the astral bodies. Just as hatha yoga strives to balance and complement the physical body with an inner awareness of energy through asana, pranayama also works to balance energies in the body.

Prana's Path

Prana does not run willy nilly through the body. It flows through the *nadi*, nerve channels. According to ancient yogic texts, there are approximately seventy-five thousand nadi in the body. The three most important nadi for the flow of prana are *sushumna, ida,* and *pingala.*

• **Sushumna** is the main channel, and it corresponds with the spinal cord.

• **Ida** is on the left of sushumna and is equated with the moon or a cooler force of energy.

• **Pingala** is opposite ida and on the right. Pingala is equated with the sun or warmer energy.

The ida and pingala are not parallel nadi, but spiral around the sushumna. Both ida and pingala correspond to the sympathetic ganglia of the

SMART DEFINITION

The Four Bodies

Yogis believe that the body is made up of different tiers or layers. There is the physical body, or the actual body; the astral, or emotional, body; the mental body, which receives and sends information and deals with thoughts; and the causal body, which is the spiritual or immortal part of man.

Source: Chakra Therapy for Personal Growth and Healing, Keith Sherwood.

spinal cord. At the base of the sushumna is the dormant energy called kundalini. Breathing practices help to uncoil the energy at the base of the spine and regulate the flow of prana through the body.

Can I Feel My Prana Flowing?

Probably not, particularly if you practice yoga intermittently or concentrate only on doing the asana. Few people report actually feeling the prana flow up their spine. Nevertheless, if you practice hatha yoga regularly, including pranayama and meditation, you will begin to feel a calm energy pervade your physical and mental being. Perhaps you suddenly feel balanced. Your body is more supple and your mind calmer. A sense of comfort and confidence prevails. Even without more sleep, you have more energy. Little things that typically bother you suddenly appear insignificant. Your intangible energy force, or prana, is percolating.

Do You Breathe Correctly?

We seldom think about breathing unless we have asthma, or are trying to huff and puff our way up a few flights of stairs, or are breathing our way through labor. We take breathing for granted, and because it is innate, who needs *breathing lessons*?

Most of us do not breathe properly. We are ineffective breathers, and over time our ineffective breathing leads to fatigue, stress, and other health problems.

Many of us breathe through our mouths. We use only the upper portion of our lungs to take in small amounts of oxygen. The diaphragm is seldom fully engaged in breathing, and we get only about a third of the oxygen our lungs need. By not filling our lungs to capacity with oxygen, we rob ourselves of vitality.

Breath and Stress

Have you ever experienced shortness of breath from anxiety, fear, or stress? If so, then you have experienced firsthand how the body, breath, and mind are connected. All these systems seem to shut down when we lose our breath. Adrenaline pumps through the body, our heartbeat accelerates, and our muscles tense up, depleting much-needed oxygen. Our breath is clearly linked to our cardiovascular, endocrine, circulatory, and digestive systems. Learning to breathe the yogi way can help us cope with stressful situations.

Pay close attention to your breath the next time you experience stressful news or get into an argument. Notice how shallow or labored your breathing becomes. You may need to gulp for air through your mouth or stop, sit down, and try to catch your breath.

Both the body and mind prosper from good breathing habits. In order to better understand the correct way to breathe, let's look at our pulmonary apparatus.

SMART MOVE

"Pranayama is the link between the mental and physical disciplines. It makes the mind calm, lucid, and steady."—Swami Vishnu Devananda, *The Sivananda Companion to Yoga*

F.Y.I.

Taking twenty minutes
a day to relax and
practice breathing tech-
niques may help
reduce hypertension
and high blood pres-
sure. Hypertension is
linked to atheroscle-
rosis, or hardening of
the arteries, and stress
is linked to hyperten-
sion. Approximately 50
million Americans
suffer from high blood
pressure, according to
the American Heart
Association.

The Breathing Cycle

The diaphragm plays a significant role in proper breathing. Situated below the rib cage, it partitions the abdominal and thoracic cavities. The diaphragm contracts and releases as we breathe. Its anatomical geography is extensive. It extends down the front of the lumbar spine where it connects with the iliopsoas muscle, a long muscle that moves along the front of the spine to the back of the pelvis into the femur. The inner spinal muscles are paramount to good postural alignment. When we breathe correctly, these muscles partner the breathing cycle to lengthen the lumbar spine. When we breathe incorrectly, the muscles do not get a significant amount of oxygen, which causes spasms or muscle tension.

The Basics of Breath

As we inhale, the diaphragm moves downward. The air is drawn down the trachea into the lungs. Simultaneously, the abdomen and rib cage expand. When we exhale, our diaphragm moves upward, compressing the lungs. This action causes the air to be expelled and the air goes back through the trachea and out the nostrils. In pranayama, you always breathe through the nose, accentuating the exhalation rather than inhalation. This cycle cleanses the lungs and eliminates toxins in the body.

Yoga's Three-Part Breathing

Yoga utilizes a three-part breathing technique. It integrates the abdominal region, lungs, and nostrils. The focus is on the following three elements:

- Inhalation

- Retention of the breath

- Exhalation

The exhalation is twice as long as the inhalation in pranayama.

Inhalation

After exhaling and clearing the lungs, inhale through the nose. The inhalation should be quiet and conscious as you fill the abdomen, lower chest, and lungs with air. When you inhale, the abdomen expands. It is after the inhalation that the breath is retained.

Retention

Retention is the next component in pranayama. It is not the same as holding your breath as you might do underwater or when you have the hiccups. In pranayama one retains the breath between inhalation and exhalation. This helps to

F.Y.I.

The Breathing Cycle of Life

Inhalation and exhalation is involuntary.

Inhalation brings oxygen to the body.

Exhalation eliminates impurities from the body.

Retention of the breath allows the mind to relax and focus.

lengthen the breathing cycle and extend the inhalation slightly. Retention creates greater respiratory capacity and concentration.

Exhalation

Exhalation is the key to yoga breathing. Breathing exercises begin with the exhalation. The more stale air exhaled out of the lungs, the more room the lungs have to inhale clean air. During exhalation, the air should be fully expelled from the abdomen and then the chest.

Abdomen! Do we really have air in our abdomens? When we breathe fully, yes. Have you ever watched an infants breathe? Notice that their little bellies rise and fall as they breathe. Infants use their abdomens, chest cavities, and nostrils to inhale and exhale. Babies are perfectly relaxed, completely unconscious of their breathing. There is nothing shallow about a baby's breath.

Expelling Impurities

The lower abdominal tract is where the body's impurities settle. Through our exhalation these impurities are eliminated. Most of us exhale unconsciously, so when we do begin to consciously exhale, it may seem like an effort to really expel all the stagnant air. Exhalation should be effortless, not forced. During exhalation you will feel the abdomen contract. Do not push the abdominal region to contract; rather, exhale gently and with awareness, letting the air push out of the abdomen. This will expel the remaining air from the lungs. The process should be naturally passive, not intentionally active.

Beginning a Basic Pranayama Practice

Pranayama will be incorporated into all the asana in hatha yoga. At the beginning of class or at the close, most hatha yoga teachers do some pranayama exercises unrelated to the asana.

Because the prana (energy) must extend through your entire body, it is best to sit with your spine erect. Your neck and head should be in a straight line, but not rigid. The classic beginning sitting pose for pranayama and meditation is the Easy Pose, or Sukhasana. (*Sukha* means "comfortable" or "joy.")

It stretches and straightens the spine, which is the fundamental conductor in pranayama, and focuses the mind.

Sukhasana (Easy Pose)

Before assuming this pose find a comfortable place on the floor. Make sure you are not too cold or too hot. The room should be quiet.

1. Sit on the floor and fold your legs, right foot just under your left leg between the calf and the foot, and left foot under your right leg between the calf and the foot. This should be comfortable, not strained. Let your knees drop only as far as comfortable.

Note: If you cannot sit on the floor or find crossing your legs even slightly uncomfortable or painful, try sitting

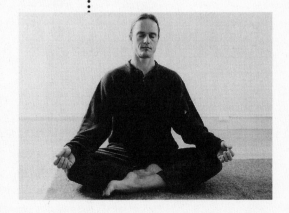

straight in a chair. If you have back problems, try putting your back against a wall for support when sitting.

2. Keep your spine erect.

3. Keep your chest erect, head forward, and shoulders back.

4. Place your hands gently on your kneecaps.

5. Close your eyes and breathe.

Mudras

A *mudra*, meaning a seal or lock, is a certain position or a definite way the fingers are held. Mudra are used in many breathing exercises and in meditation. Vishnu mudra is the mudra used for basic pranayama.

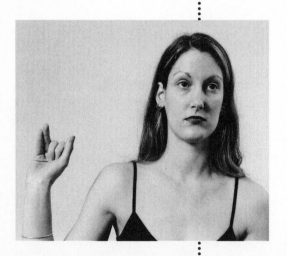

Vishnu Mudra Position

With your right hand, extend the thumb, ring finger, and little finger, then fold the middle and index fingers toward your palm. Your left hand remains inactive at your side or on your left knee.

Vishnu mudra may seem kind of strange, and maybe you feel a little uncomfortable blocking off your nostrils with your fingers in the name of breathing. You don't have to do this in a restaurant or phone booth; save it for yoga class or the privacy of your own home. The best way to acquaint yourself with this basic mudra is to practice with the Single Nostril Breathing Exercise (see page 49).

Qualities of Pranayama

There are three elements or qualities of pranayama. They are the following:

- **Desha**, which refers to where you are focused mentally

- **Kala**, the equal ratio in pranayama between the inhalation, exhalation, and retention

- **Samkhya**, which refers to the pattern of breathing or length of time spent practicing pranayama

Breathing Exercises

The great advantage to practicing pranayama is that it revitalizes the body as well as the mind. It leads to a sense of well-being and clarity. The effects of pranayama can be physical as well as psychological, and it is always advisable to have a yoga teacher instruct you with the breathing practices before adopting them on your own. Advanced pranayama practices are powerful tools for raising energy and should always be guided by a knowledgeable teacher.

SMART SOURCES

Want to know more about breathing, and not just for yoga? Check out Donna Farhi's *The Breathing Book*, a comprehensive work on the right—and wrong—way to breathe.

1. Warming Up the Breath

Here's a simple exercise to help you understand and feel how you breathe.

1. Lie on the floor on your back.

2. Relax the body and breathe normally for a minute or two.

3. Consciously begin to get in touch with how you breathe. Are you breathing through your nose or mouth? Is your breathing easy or difficult?

4. Now place your hand on your abdomen and breathe.

Do you feel the abdomen move up and down with each inhalation and exhalation? Can you feel the air travel up into your chest?

Practice this until you get in touch with your breathing rhythms. If you would like, try this exercise for a week and keep track of the difference between your breathing awareness the first day through the last day.

2. Full-Breath Exercise

Here's a breathing exercise that will help you physically feel the fullness of your breath.

1. Sit in the Easy Pose and place one hand on your abdomen and the other hand slightly above it on your rib cage.

2. As you breathe in, feel the abdomen expand with one hand and the air move up through your lungs with the other hand.

3. Exhale and feel your chest move in slightly and notice your abdomen contract.

3. Single-Nostril Breathing Exercise

1. Sitting in the Easy Pose, make the Vishnu mudra with your right hand.

2. Bring it to your right nostril and close off the right nostril with your thumb.

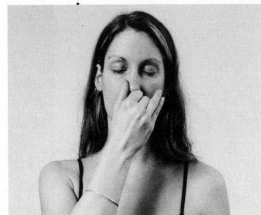

3. Inhale through the left nostril.

4. Hold for the count of four and exhale.

5. Repeat five to eight times.

6. Then using the right hand, which is still forming the Vishnu mudra, close off the left nostril with the ring and little fingers.

7. Inhale through the right nostril and count to four and exhale.

8. Repeat five to eight times.

4. Nadi Sodhana (Alternate-Nostril Breathing Exercise)

This is one of the very first breathing exercises taught in a yoga class. *Nadi,* as we discussed in chapter 3, are like nerve channels for the passage of prana, and *sodhana* means "to cleanse." This is a natural extension of the Single-Nostril Breathing Exercise and a good way to begin or end the day. It purifies the nadis, and calms and helps focus the mind.

1. Sit comfortably in the Easy Pose.

2. Make the Vishnu mudra position with your right hand.

3. Inhale through the left nostril to the count of four.

4. Close the nostrils and hold the breath to a count between twelve and sixteen. You may need to work up to this count.

5. Pinching off the left nostril, exhale through your right nostril to the count of eight.

6. Inhale through your right nostril to the count of four.

7. Close the nostrils and hold the breath to the count of sixteen.

8. Still pinching off the right nostril, exhale through the left nostril to the count of eight.

9. Repeat four to eight times.

10. Breathe normally.

5. Kapalabhati (The Skull Shining Breath)

Kapalabhati is a slightly more advanced breathing exercise, but it is a natural progression from the Alternate-Nostril Breathing Exercise. It is a good purifying practice and is invigorating.

Kapalabhati is a series of rapid exhalations and inhalations followed by a retention of the breath. The air pumps in and out of your lungs, and it takes a little practice to obtain the correct rhythm.

Kapalabhati rids the lungs of stale air and opens the way for fresh oxygen. With practice you can work up to thirty, forty, or fifty pumps per series.

1. Begin with an exhalation. To exhale, contract the abdominal muscles, sharply forcing the air out of the lungs. Exhalations are brief and active. You will be able to hear the exhalation in this exercise.

2. To inhale, relax the abdominal muscles your the lungs will fill with air. Inhalation is longer than exhalation and significantly silent compared to exhalation.

3. Allow the movements to cause the diaphragm to move up and down.

WHAT MATTERS, WHAT DOESN'T

What Matters

• Practicing breathing in a quiet place without background noise.

• Understanding that pranayama takes some practice.

• Not retaining your breath if you feel short of breath or uncomfortable. Breathe naturally.

• That you consult your doctor before embarking on breathing exercises if you are sick or have respiratory problems.

What Doesn't

• That you retain the breath for a long time.

• That it takes some time to learn to breathe efficiently.

• That you've spent your life breathing inefficiently.

• That you can't explain pranayama to your spouse or friends.

4. Practice three rounds of Kapalabhati with twenty pumps in each round. Air will be pushed through your nostrils on the exhalation and you will hear it. It sounds as if you are trying to sniff something out of your nostrils, such as a bee or bug. Although the inhalation is quieter, the combination of the two is rapid. After each round, take a few deep breaths before starting the next round.

6. Bhastrika (Bellows Breath)

The last pranayama exercise is Bhastrika, or the Bellows Breath. Just as a bellows heats up the fire, Bhastrika heats up the body. It helps the prana flow freely through the spine. You might want to keep a tissue close by; this is a good sinus cleanser and a natural decongestant.

1. Sit in the Easy Pose.

2. Exhale deeply and sharply. This action pulls the abdominal muscles inward.

3. Breathe rapidly through the nose with sharp, deliberate deep movements. The inhalation is reflexive, you won't need to think about it. You will feel the action of this movement in the base of your throat. Don't hold your breath between breaths.

4. Begin with five rounds and work up to ten. Between rounds, hold your breath for a few seconds.

By practicing one or two of these breathing exercises you will begin to see and feel how your breathing reflects on your daily activities. Full yogic breathing leads to a calmer state of mind.

In the following chapter you will marvel at how flawlessly interdependent the body and the breath work together when performing asana.

THE BOTTOM LINE

The ultimate goal in pranayama is to focus the mind. In hatha yoga, the postures utilize the most basic pranayama practices. When practicing asana, we pay attention to our breath and how our breathing affects the asana. There is a clear connection between the mind and the body, breathing and movement. As the asana strengthen the body, pranayama helps to focus the mind. Your rate of breathing and your state of mind are inseparable.

CHAPTER 4

·······················

The Asana

There is a wealth of benefits that you will experience when you practice the asana. While every school of yoga has its own approach to the asana, the results are the same. The asana nourish the body, mind, and spirit, intimately connecting the triad to wellness.

The Benefits of Asana

With asana, stretching and alignment of the body are a given. But both the body and the mind obtain a constellation of benefits, such as energy and serenity; balance and control; and focus and strength, to mention just a few. Your entire body—from your adrenal and endocrine glands to your heart to your muscles, ligaments, and joints—will benefit from practicing asana.

Some of the physical benefits of doing asana are the following:

• Create spinal suppleness

• Tone muscles

• Tone glands

• Tone internal organs

• Tone joints

• Strengthen the musculoskeletal system

• Enhance flexibility

- Enhance balance

- Help with agility and coordination

The Practice of Asana

Asana strives to strike a balance, to create strength and flexibility, or sthira and sukha. *Sukha* means "comfortable" and *sthira* means "steady," and in asana one should strive for both. Some of us start out with a little more sthira than sukha, or vice versa. Of course, everyone will have different limitations in a beginning hatha yoga class. No two bodies are alike.

Start slowly with your asana routine. Keep in mind that in order to obtain the maximum benefits, you will need to practice. It's best to practice the asana daily, and it is vital that you practice the asana correctly.

Hatha yoga requires some space. The best place to practice asana is in a quiet area or empty room, on a folded mat or carpeted floor. There should be no music or chatter or competition. The atmosphere ought to be relaxed. It's best to wear loose-fitting clothing, nothing restricting, and practice in bare feet. Asana should be performed on an empty stomach.

The Sequence of Asana

When you practice hatha yoga, it is important to do the asana in sequence. The word hatha is made up of two words: *ha*, which is "sun," and *tha*, which is "moon." One is the masculine energy, the other

F.Y.I.

The very first principle of yoga is to get in touch with your body. How does it feel? Is it tense or relaxed? Do you have muscle cramps, stiff joints, or malaise? Do you have a general sense of discomfort or do you feel pretty good these days? Does your back hurt or do you suffer from headaches? Take some time with your personal body scan and make mental notes of what is going on in your body.

is the feminine energy, both of which exist in every one of us. Practicing asana unites these elements.

Each asana will either augment or counterbalance the prior asana. Each series of asana would be counterbalanced, such as the forward bending series being followed by a series of backward bending poses. If you do an asana that stretches or works one side of your body, you will always repeat the asana on the other side of the body. Every pose offers unique benefits for the various systems in your body.

Anatomy of an Asana

There are three stages to each pose or asana.

1. Getting into the pose

2. Holding the pose

3. Coming out of the pose

In asana, you gently stretch into the pose and hold it for several seconds. You never stop breathing; it's important to breathe easily and with awareness. When the breath is used properly, it helps the stretch into the pose and allows you to hold a pose longer. Release the pose and gently come out of it and rest before starting another asana. Always come out of a pose if you feel any discomfort.

Depending on your yoga teacher, style, and level, poses are held for different time intervals. Some may be held for thirty seconds, sixty seconds, or three to five minutes. This book does not offer a suggested length of time to hold the asana.

A caveat: No matter what your level, never force or hold an asana to the point of discomfort.

The Asana Illustrated

Several of the asana or poses in this book are beginning poses; others are intermediate or advanced. Most of the poses can be modified for all levels. The asana in this chapter are grouped by their characteristics and/or basic movements, not by the sequence in which they would necessarily be taught in a class. The illustrated asana groupings are the following:

- Standing Poses

- Sitting Poses

- Forward Bending Poses

- Reclining or Supine Poses

- Backward Bending Poses

- Inverted Poses

- Twisting Poses

- Balancing Poses

- Relaxation Pose

- Poses for Women (But Not Exclusively)

The chapter concludes with Surya Namaskara, the Sun Salutation, a series of twelve contiguous, flowing poses that are the foundation for many other yoga poses.

No matter which pose or group of poses you choose to practice, start with the most elementary.

The first lesson of yoga is how to stand. Let's begin with the standing poses.

Standing Poses

The standing poses teach the basics of alignment, concentration, and coordination. They help establish a foundation for many of the other poses. Standing poses should be part of a daily practice. One typically jumps into these poses, but you need not jump into a pose to obtain the benefits. If you have back or knee injuries or are pregnant, do not jump into the pose. A number of the standing poses are invigorating. Standing poses can be strenuous, and some are more so than others. Always come out of a pose if you feel fatigued or unsteady.

1. Tadasana (The Mountain Pose)

Many of the poses in yoga are named after animals, birds, or elements, such as the most basic pose, Tadasana. *Tada* means "mountain," and *asana*, "posture." Just as a mountain symbolizes steadiness and stability, Tadasana is the steady, stable pose that sets the tone for all the other poses.

Most yoga classes begin with Tadasana. The pose roots the body to the ground, permitting it to grow or to stand tall. Think of it as a kind of natural position between your feet, which are firmly planted on the earth or ground, and your head, which reaches toward the sky, connecting everything in between. Good posture is paramount in yoga, and Tadasana is your first lesson or pose on posture.

Benefits: Improves posture; balances the body; focuses the mind.

Instructions:

1. Stand with your feet together or slightly apart. The weight of your body should be evenly distributed between the toes, balls, and heels of your feet.

2. Keep your knees as straight as possible without locking them. Pay attention to your stomach, but do not suck it in or let it sag.

3. Keep your shoulders and arms relaxed and straight. Arms remain at your sides.

4. Your head should look straight ahead. Do not strain your neck muscles.

5. Relax your eyes and try to organize the body from head to toe as you breathe. Your breathing should be clear and strong as it moves through you.

6. Your inhalation and exhalation should be natural, giving you a sense of relaxation.

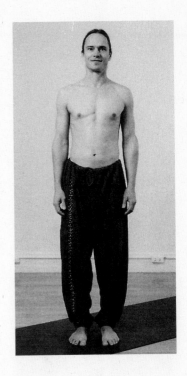

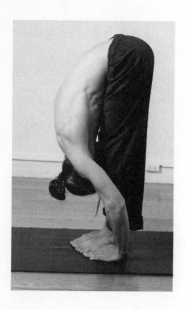

2. Uttanasana (Standing Forward–Bending Pose)

Translation: *Ut* refers to a "particle of doubt or deliberation"; *tan,* "to stretch or to extend."

Benefits: Tones abdominal organs; soothes the mind.

Instructions:

1. Stand in Tadasana.

2. Stretch arms overhead, palms facing forward.

3. As you exhale, gently bend forward.

4. Place your fingers or hands on the floor on each side of your feet and move your head toward your knees. Breathe into the position.

5. Exhale as you reverse the pose to come out of it.

Note: You may be able to stretch your fingers only as far as your knees or abdomen. Beginners should not push the stretch further than is comfortable. Stretch only as far as you can. With practice, flexibility will increase.

3. Trikonasana (Triangle Pose)

Translation: *Tri* means "three"; *kona,* "angle."

Benefits: Tones and stretches leg, hip, and back muscles.

Instructions:

1. Spread the legs about 3 or 4 feet apart.

2. Inhale and stretch the arms out to the sides.

3. Exhaling, extend the right arm upward, stretching over to the left side of the body, and place the left palm against your leg.

4. Your head should be looking upward toward the stretched right arm. Be careful not to bend forward; aim for a triangle position. Stretch only as far as you can. Breathe into the pose.

5. Inhale and come back to center.

6. Repeat on the opposite side.

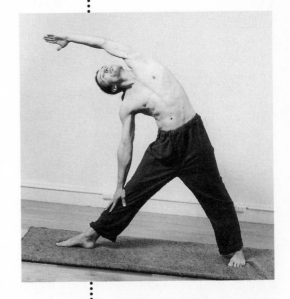

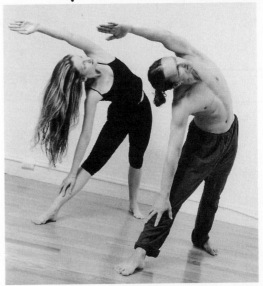

4. Virabhadrasana (The Warrior Pose)

Translation: *Virabhadra* means "warrior."

Benefits: Relieves stiffness in the back and shoulders; strengthens legs.

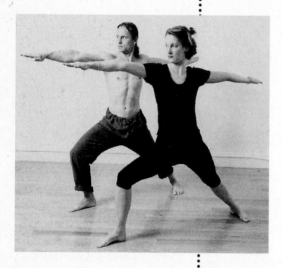

Instructions:

1. From Tadasana, jump and spread the legs about 3 or 4 feet apart.

2. Stretch the arms to the side in a line, right palm facing downward, left palm facing up.

3. Turn the right foot 90 degrees and the left foot slightly to the right.

4. Exhale and bend the right knee. The right thigh should be parallel to the floor.

5. Keep the left leg stretched and the knee in line.

6. Stretch both arms, then turn the face to the right and line the eyes with the right palm.

7. Stretch thoroughly and breathe.

8. Repeat for the opposite side.

Note: This pose is strenuous. Avoid it if you have a heart condition or are not very strong.

Sitting Poses

The sitting poses are good poses to align the spine, steady the body, and focus concentration. They are considered calming poses.

5. Sukhasana (Easy Pose)

Translation: *Sukha* means "comfortable" or "joy."

Benefits: Sukhasana is the basic pose for sitting and relaxation and is the classic pose for beginning meditation. It stretches the spine and focuses the mind.

Instructions:

1. Sit on the floor and fold the legs, right foot just under your left leg between the calf and the foot, and left foot under your right leg between the calf and the foot. This should be comfortable, not strained. Let your knees drop only as far as comfortable.

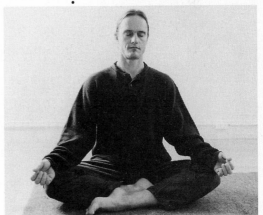

Note: If you cannot sit on the floor or find crossing your legs even slightly uncomfortable or painful, try sitting straight in a chair. If you have back problems, try putting your back against a wall for support when sitting.

2. Keep your spine erect.

3. Keep your chest erect, head forward, and shoulders back.

4. Place your hands gently on your kneecaps.

5. Close your eyes and breathe.

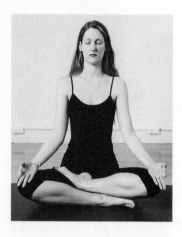

6. Padmasana (Lotus Pose)

Translation: *Padma* means "lotus."

Benefits: Straightens spine; calms mind; increases concentration.

Instructions:

1. Sit erect. Spread your legs in front of you into a V shape.

2. Bend the right leg as you bring the foot in toward the body and place it on the top of the opposite thigh.

3. Bring in the left foot the same way and place it on the top of the opposite thigh.

4. For the Half Lotus, called Ardha Padmasana, fold the left foot on the opposite thigh, and fold the right foot on the floor under the opposite leg.

Note: The lotus pose requires flexibility and should never be forced. Many people who have practiced yoga for years never acquire the flexibility for a full lotus. Pay attention to your knees in the lotus.

7. Bhaddha Konasana
(Bound Eagle Pose; Butterfly Pose)

Translation: *Bhadda* is "to restrain" and *kona* means "angle."

Benefits: Aids pelvis, abdomen, and back.

Instructions:

1. Sit with the spine erect and your legs spread in a V shape.

2. Bring the heels of your feet together in front of you. Allow the knees to fall comfortably toward the floor.

3. Clasp your hands around your feet, keeping the spine erect as your upper torso eases forward. This pose naturally stretches the spine and inner thighs.

  Note: Do this pose with care if you have bad knees. Never force the knees downward.

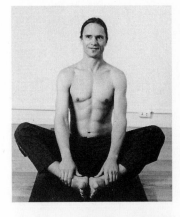

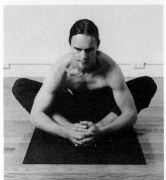

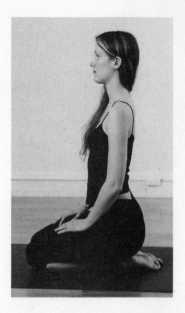

8. Vajrasana (Kneeling Pose)

Translation: *Vajra* means "thunderbolt."

Benefits: Aligns spinal column; calms and focuses the mind.

Instructions:

1. Sit back on your heels with your knees bent under you.

2. Keep your spine erect, and place your hands on your knees. Breathe.

Note: Avoid if you have knee problems or knee injuries.

9. Seated Chair Stretch

Benefits: Good for an upper body stretch; relieves muscle tension.

Instructions:

1. Sit on the edge of a chair in your home or office. Do not use a swiveling chair.

2. Put your left hand behind your back, the palm turned away from your back. Stretch the right arm upward.

3. Take the upward extended hand and reach behind your back to grasp the left hand. Hold and breathe into the stretch.

4. Repeat for the opposite side.

Note: One side of your body will probably be more flexible than the other side. The stretch is difficult and you may not be able to reach the other hand. Stretch only as far as you can. Use a handkerchief or a towel in the upward stretched arm and allow the hand behind your back to grasp it. This will aid the stretch.

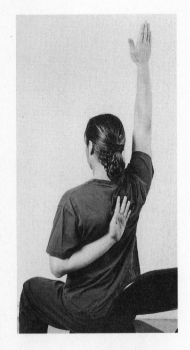

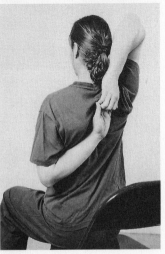

Forward Bending Poses

Seated forward bends are introspective and calm the mind. Some of the poses are more vigorous than others. A few of the poses are considered good restorative poses. All tone the abdominals.

10. Paschinottanasana (Seated Forward Bend)

Translation: *Paschima* means "back side of the body."

Benefits: Tones abdominal organs; stretches entire spine.

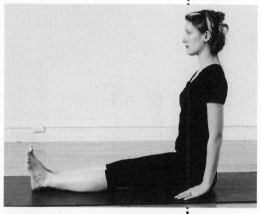

Instructions:

1. Sit on the floor with your legs together and stretched in front of you.

2. With your spine erect and head looking forward, inhale as you stretch your arms overhead with your hands touching, palms facing legs.

3. As you exhale, bend forward, hands stretching toward the feet and head stretching toward the knees.

4. You may not be able to stretch this far; go only as far as you can. Breathe into the position. Inhale and slowly come up back to the beginning position.

11. Janu-Shirshasana (Head-to-Knee Pose)

Translation: *Janu* is "knee"; *shirsha* is "head."

Benefits: Tones liver and spleen; aids digestion; stretches spine.

Instructions:

1. Sit on the floor with legs stretched in front. Bend your left leg and bring your left foot to the inner thigh of your right leg.

2. Keep your right leg stretched in front.

3. Inhale and bring your hands overhead, touching, palms facing forward.

4. Exhaling, bend toward the outstretched leg.

5. Clasp your feet with both hands and bring your head down as far as you can toward your right knee. Breathe into the position. Release, inhale, and come up, then alternate legs and sides.

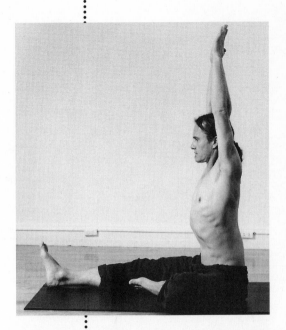

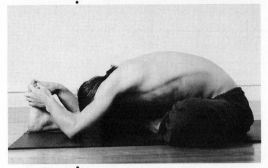

12. Upavista Konasana (Open Angle Pose)

Translation: *Upavista* means "seated"; *kona* is "angle."

Benefits: This pose stretches the hamstrings and back.

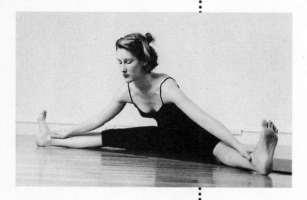

Instructions:

1. Sit on the floor with your legs stretched out in a V shape.

2. Keep your back and upper torso erect. As you exhale, gently bend forward, stretching the right hand toward the right foot and the left hand toward the left foot; stretch to grasp the toes.

3. Breathe into the pose and release.

Reclining or Supine Poses

The reclining poses are considered relaxing and less strenuous. They are helpful poses for relieving tension and fatigue and are beneficial during menstruation.

13. Savasana (Corpse Pose; Relaxation Pose)

Translation: *Sava* means "corpse."

Benefits: Relaxes and replenishes the body, mind, and spirit. This is a good pose to do between asana and again at the completion of your practice. Savasana is the pose for yoga *nidra,* which means "sleep." Yoga nidra is the final relaxation at the end of many yoga classes.

Instructions:
1. Lie flat on your back on a blanket or mat. Keep your hands by your sides, palms up. Legs are parallel, feet slightly apart.

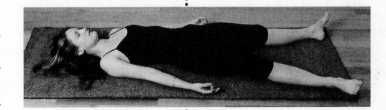

2. Close your eyes. Begin to breathe slowly and deliberately. Concentrate on the exhalation.

3. Relax everything from your face to your toes.

14. Supta-Padangusthasana (Reclining Single-Leg Raise)

Translation: *Supta* means "sleeping"; *padagnustha* means "the big toe."

Benefits: Strengthens abdominal muscles and stretches hamstrings.

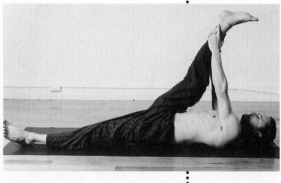

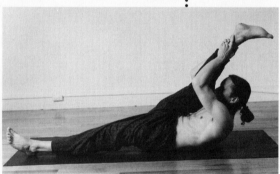

Instructions:

1. Lie on your back, making sure your back is flat on the floor.

2. Keep your arms at your side. Inhaling, raise your right leg as high as possible without bending your knees.

3. Keep your left leg straight on the floor. Place your hands around your right ankle. Beginners may not be able to reach the ankle; more advanced yoga practitioners or limber individuals may be able to reach farther up to the foot. Go only as far as you can without discomfort.

4. Breathe into the pose. Exhale as you lower your right leg. Repeat for the alternate leg.

15. Apanasana (Wind-Relieving Pose)

Translation: *Apana* means "lower abdomen."

Benefits: Massages abdominal organs and releases gas from the intestines.

Instructions:

1. Lie on your back on the floor and bring your knees toward your chest.

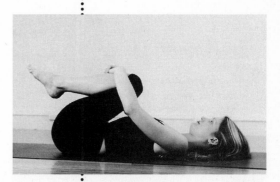

2. Wrap your arms around your legs, and press your legs toward your chest.

3. Bring your head toward your knees. Hold the pose.

4. Exhale and release your legs. You can also gently rock back and forth in this position to massage the spinal area.

Backward Bending Poses

Backward-bending poses energize and open the body, particularly the chest cavity. They strengthen the upper body, increase spinal flexibility, and stimulate the nervous system. Backward-bending poses should not be done if you have knee injuries, high blood pressure, heart disease, or if you are pregnant. You should rest in the Corpse Pose after these poses to replenish your energy before moving on.

16. Dhanurasana (Bow Pose)

Translation: *Dhanu* means "bow."

Benefits: Improves spinal elasticity; tones the abdominal organs; increases vitality.

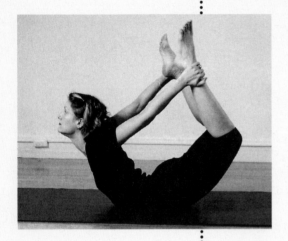

Instructions:

1. Lie on your stomach, face down, forehead on the floor.

2. Bend the knees. Keeping your head forward, reach back with your right arm and hold your right ankle; with your left arm reach back and hold your left ankle.

3. The weight will be balanced on your abdomen.

4. Exhale and gently pull your legs up by raising your knees off the floor as you lift your chest slightly.

5. Lift your head and look straight ahead. You may rock back and forth in this position. Breathe.

Note: This pose has many stages. In the beginning you may be able to hold your calves, not your ankles, or you may not be able to raise your legs or chest off the floor.

17. Bhujangasana (Cobra)

Translation: *Bhujanga* means "serpent" or "snake."

Benefits: Provides good backward spinal stretch; tones abdominal organs.

Instructions:
Note: This pose should be stretched vertebra by vertebra.

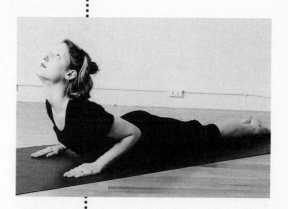

1. Lie on your stomach, legs together.

2. Arms should be at your side near your shoulder with your palms down.

3. Rest your forehead on the floor. Inhale, then slowly bring your head up in sequence of forehead, nose, and chin.

4. Now lift your hands and use your upper back muscles to slowly arch backward. Do not push up on your hands; you should be able to do this without your hands.

5. Inhale and raise up a little more. Legs should be straight and on the ground. Hold for the count of three, then exhale and slowly roll down.

18. Setu Bandhasana (Bridge Pose)

Translation: *Setu* is "bridge."

Benefits: Stretches abdominal and lumbar spine muscles.

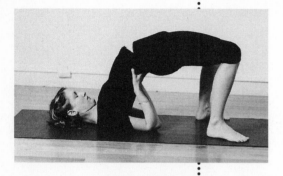

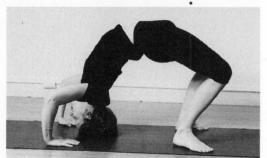

Instructions:

1. Lie down flat on your back with your knees bent, feet together. Arms should be at your sides.

2. Place your hands on your lower back and lift your hips up as high as possible. Your head, neck, and shoulders should remain on the floor. Arch.

3. From this pose, if you are flexible you may arch up into the Wheel Pose (see bottom photo).

Note: The Bridge Pose is used when coming out of the Shoulder Stand (see page 83); however, to come from the Shoulder Stand into the Bridge you must have a flexible back.

19. Matsyasana (Fish Pose)

Translation: *Matsya* means "fish."

Benefits: This is the counterpose for the Shoulder Stand and always follows it. It opens the chest, tones the nerves in the neck and back, aids in deep breathing, and expands lung capacity.

Instructions:

1. Lie down on your back. Your legs should be straight with your feet together. Place your hands at your sides, palms down and under your buttocks.

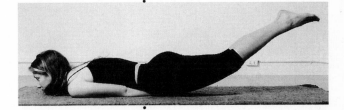

2. Press down on your elbows, inhale, and arch your back.

3. The crown of your head should be on the floor. Exhale.

4. Breathe deeply into this pose and keep your legs and lower body relaxed.

5. To come out of the pose, lift your head and place it gently back down, release your arms, and relax.

Note: Stay in this pose half the amount of time that you stayed in the Shoulder Stand.

20. Salabhasana (Locust Pose)

Translation: *Salabha* means "locust."

Benefits: Strengthens the abdomen, lower back, and legs; aids digestion.

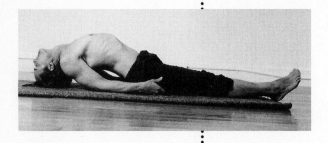

Instructions:

1. Lie on your stomach with your chin on the floor.

2. Stretch your arms under your body so that you are lying on them.

3. Take a few deep breaths in this position. Inhale and raise your right leg. Breathe into the pose.

4. Exhale and lower your right leg.

5. Repeat with the opposite leg, then repeat by lifting both legs.

Note: This pose is strenuous and you should do it with caution if you have lower back pain. Lift only one leg at a time in the beginning.

Inverted Poses

Inverted poses reverse gravity and supply fresh blood to the head and heart. They are considered revitalizing and tone internal organs, stimulate the brain, and improve circulation. But note this caveat: inverted poses should not be done if you are pregnant or menstruating or if you have high blood pressure, headaches, coronary problems, or neck or spinal injuries. These are fairly advanced poses, and you should relax between each pose.

21. Adho Mukha Shvanasana (Downward-Facing Dog Pose)

Translation: *Adho mukha* means "to face downward."

Benefits: Stretches and releases tension in the upper spine and neck; strengthens and stretches legs and arms.

Instructions:

1. Begin on your hands and knees.

2. Lift your tailbone up and bring your knees off of the floor.

3. Stretch your shoulders and head downward.

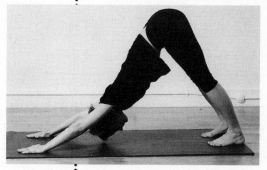

4. With bent knees, work to bring your heels to the floor and straighten your legs.

5. Keep your hips lifted, and stretch. Your weight should be evenly distributed on your hands and heels, just like a dog who stretches after a good nap.

6. The focus in this asana is on stretching your back, not on getting your heels to the floor. Breathe.

7. To come out of the pose, go down on all fours.

Note: Be careful not to stress the Achilles tendon when pressing the heels to the floor if you are not flexible or have not sufficiently warmed up.

22. Halasana (Plow Pose)

Translation: *Hala* means "plow."

Benefits: Aids spine and hip flexibility; nourishes the spinal nerves; strengthens the back.

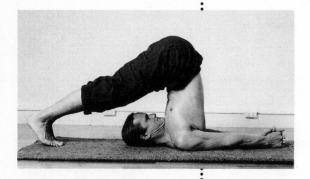

Instructions:
1. Lie down on the floor on a blanket or a mat.

2. Place your arms straight at your sides with your palms down and legs together.

3. Inhale, then raise your legs up.

4. Exhale, then inhale and bring your hips off the floor. Put your hands on your lower back for support, keeping your elbows close to your body.

5. Without bending your knees, exhale and bring your legs down behind your head, trying to touch your feet to the floor. Breathe.

6. You may not be able to touch the floor. Bring your legs only as far back as comfortable. To release, roll out of the pose onto your back.

23. Sarvangasana (Shoulder Stand)

Translation: *Sarvanga* means "all parts of the body."

Benefits: Rejuvenates entire body; stretches neck and upper spine; stimulates the thyroid and parathyroid glands. The Shoulder Stand is considered the queen of the poses.

Instructions:

1. Lie on the floor with your legs together.

2. Place your hands, palms down, next to your side. Inhale, push down on your hands, and raise your legs straight above you.

3. Lift your hips off the floor and bring the legs up and over the head at an angle.

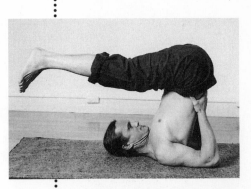

4. Exhale, bend your arms, place your palms on your spine, and, supporting your body, gently push your back up. Keep your arms as close to your body as possible. Breathe slowly and deeply.

5. Work to straighten the torso.

6. Roll out of the pose slowly, lowering your legs to an angle over your head. Place your hands, palms down, behind you.

7. Exhaling, continue to roll out until your entire body is resting on the floor. Relax.

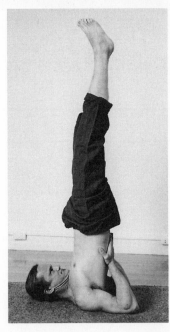

Note: This pose is not advised for individuals who have a neck injury or high blood pressure or who are menstruating or pregnant.

24. Shirshasana (Head Stand)

Translation: *Shirsha* means "head."

Benefits: Shirshasana is considered the king of all asana. Its benefits are numerous, from reversing gravity to aiding circulation. This pose also improves memory, concentration, and sensory acuity.

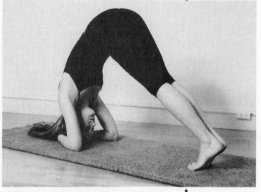

Instructions:

1. The focus in this asana is balancing on the forearms and elbows, not the head.

2. Kneel down with your elbows touching the floor. Rest your weight on your elbows.

3. Fold your hands together, palms facing you. Keep your fingers interlocked and place them in front of you with your elbows on the floor. This is your base.

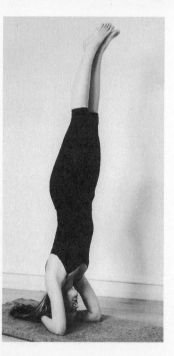

4. Place the back of your head inside your clasped hands with the crown of your head on the floor.

5. Straighten your knees and raise your hips. Do not bend your knees, but walk your feet as close to your head as possible.

6. Bring your hips back so that your neck is not bent.

7. Concentrating, bend your knees and lift your feet from the floor. Pause, then slowly, keeping your knees bent, lift them toward the sky.

8. Slowly straighten your legs. The body's weight should be on the forearms, not the head.

9. To release, reverse the position. Bring your knees down to your chest, then to the floor. Kneel down as you did in the beginning of the pose and go into the Child's Pose (see page 92, Mudhasana—the counterpose for the headstand.

Note: Even if you just do the preparation pose, without actually completing the headstand, there are numerous benefits.

Twisting Poses

Twisting poses energize the body and increase range of motion and spinal flexibility. They are good poses for relieving neck and shoulder stiffness.

25. Ardha Matsyendransana (Half Spinal Twist)

Translation: The name comes from the yogic sage Matsyendra.

Benefits: Rotates the spine; tones spinal nerves; improves the nervous system; aids digestion.

Instructions:
1. Sit on the floor with your legs stretched out in front.

2. Bend your right knee up and move your right leg over to the outside of

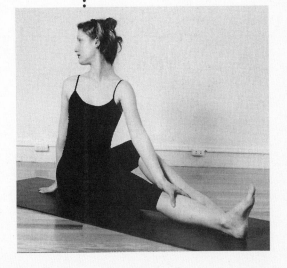

your left leg, near your knee. Place your right heel and foot on the floor. Keep the spine erect.

3. Stretch both arms out to the side and bring the left arm to the outside of the right knee; twisting to the right, place your right hand on the floor behind you.

4. Exhaling, twist as far as possible as you look over your shoulder.

5. Do not lift your shoulders.

6. To come out of the pose, gently twist back to the front of your body.

7. Repeat for the opposite side.

Note: Twist only as far as you comfortably can.

26. Bharadvajasana (Chair Spinal Twist)

Translation: Bharadvaja is the name of a sage.

Benefits: Alleviates tension in the spine; stretches the spinal muscles.

Instructions:

1. Sit on the edge of your chair. Your spine should be erect.

2. Reach around with your left arm and place it on the back of the chair or behind you.

3. With your right arm reach across the front of your body and twist, turning the upper torso to the left. Breathe and release.

4. Repeat for the opposite side.

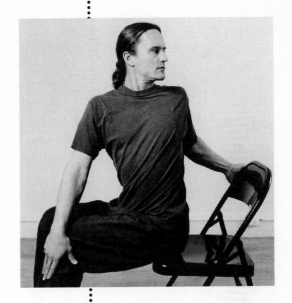

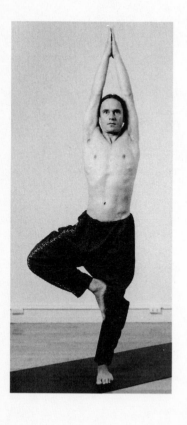

Balancing Poses

Balancing poses develop agility, concentration, and strength. You should rest after each of these poses.

27. Vrksasana (Tree Pose)

Translation: *Vrksa* means "tree."

Benefits: Stretches entire body; tones leg muscles; helps develop balance and concentration.

Instructions:
Practice the tree in stages.

1. Begin in Tadasana (standing pose) with your hands in front of you in a prayer position.

2. Balance on one leg, then slide the opposite foot up the inside of the balancing leg to the ankle or calf.

3. When you are comfortable, continue to slide the foot to the knee of the standing leg.

4. Concentrate and raise both arms over your head, palms together.

28. Natarajasana Variation (King Dancer Pose)

Translation: Nataraja is one of the names of the Hindu god Siva, the Cosmic Dancer.

Benefits: Increases strength, suppleness, and balance.

Instructions:

1. Stand straight, in Tadasana.

2. Inhale as you bend your left leg back, grasping the foot or ankle with your left hand. Exhale.

3. Balance yourself, and on the next inhalation raise and extend the right arm, keeping it near your head.

4. Balance and breathe.

5. Repeat on the other side.

Note: This is an advanced balancing pose.

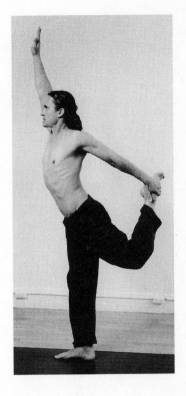

29. Mayurasana (The Peacock Pose)

Translation: *Mayura* means "peacock."

Benefits: Aids concentration; good for digestion; strengthens arm muscles.

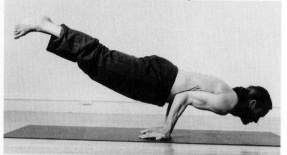

Instructions:

1. Kneel on the floor. Sit back on your heels with your knees apart.

2. Place your palms on the floor inverted. Fingers should be facing you.

3. Bend forward, keeping your arms up to the elbow straight, and place the top of your head on the floor. Your elbows should be parallel, pressing into the upper part of your abdomen.

4. Stretch your legs back, keeping the knees off the floor and the feet together. Weight ought to be on your toes, hands, and head.

5. Lift your head. Inhale and gently shift forward on your arms, lifting the toes up and balancing on your hands.

6. The legs should remain straight. Breathe into the pose and hold as long as you can. Exhale and release, coming down on your toes.

Note: This is an advanced, strenuous pose. If you have weak wrists or little strength, this will not be the pose for you. As in all poses, you can do the preparation part of the pose and still gain the benefits, without actually doing the entire pose.

30. Eka Pada Rajakapotasana (One-Legged Dove Pose)

Translation: *Eka* is "one"; *pada*, "leg"; and *kapota*, "dove."

Benefits: Expands the lungs; stretches the abdominal muscles and the spine.

Instructions:

1. Exhaling, bend the left knee so that the foot is on the floor, heel toward the groin or thigh. The left knee should be on the floor.

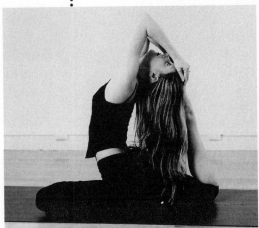

2. Inhale and take the right leg and bring it back behind your body; stretch it behind you on the floor.

3. Rest your hands on the floor in front of you and breathe. On your exhalation, take your hands over your head. Simultaneously, bend your left leg at the knee toward your head, griping your left foot with your hands. Exhale, and stretch your head back to touch your foot. Rest your head on your foot.

4. Stretch and breathe into the pose.

Note: This is an advanced pose and requires strength and flexibility. It should not be done by those with bad knees or by beginners.

Relaxation Pose

This pose is used throughout asana and is a great restorative, restful pose. Go into this pose whenever you feel fatigue or want to rest.

31. Mudhasana (Child's Pose)

Translation: *Mudha* means "silly" or "childish."

Benefits: This pose relaxes the body between other poses and is considered a nice rejuvenating, gentle, nurturing pose. Good for relief of back pain and to help balance the mind.

Instructions:

1. Kneeling down, sit on the back of your heels.

2. Bend forward and bring your forehead to the ground; bring your arms around your sides toward the back.

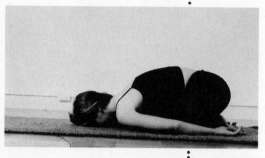

3. Sink into the pose and breathe deeply and fully. Relax. Keep the spine stretched.

4. Another version of this pose is to stretch your arms in front of you instead of behind you.

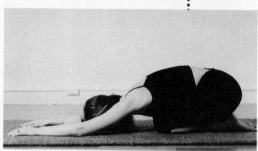

Poses for Women (But Not Exclusively)

While anyone can do these poses and obtain the benefits, they are especially good for women during pregnancy, menses, or menopause. These poses are good for opening the pelvic area and relieving tension.

32. Pelvic Tilt

Benefits: This pose helps to strengthen the uterus and pelvic region. It is also good for relieving back pain and for menstruation.

Instructions:

1. Lie on your back, arms to your sides, palms down.

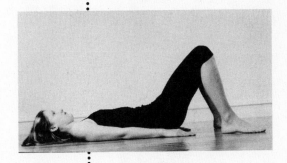

2. Inhale and slowly and ever so gently, tilt your pelvis upward, slightly off the floor. Hold for a few seconds and breathe.

3. Exhaling, gently release, placing the pelvis back on the ground.

4. Repeat.

33. Bidalasana (The Cat Pose)

Translation: *Bidala* means "cat."

Benefits: Strengthens abdomen; alleviates back-aches. This is a good all-around pose and can be done during pregnancy.

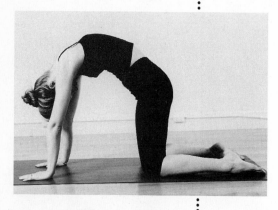

Instructions:
1. Get down on all fours and look straight ahead. Make sure your arms are even with your shoulders.

2. Exhale and arch upward, head bent, like a cat when frightened. The lower back will be flat, the head looking down toward the abdomen. Breathe naturally.

3. Inhale and arch downward, curving the lower back.

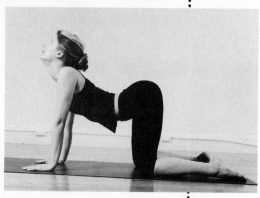

4. Lift your head up and breathe naturally.

5. Relax and repeat six times.

34. Malasana (Squatting Pose)

Translation: *Mala* means "garland."

Benefits: The is a wonderful pose to open the pelvic area to prepare for birth.

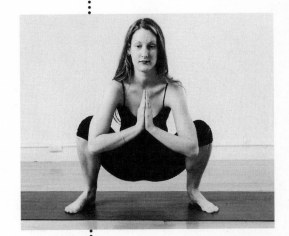

Instructions:

1. Stand in Tadasana and bring your hands into the prayer position.

2. Spread your legs about three feet apart and slowly go into a squatting position.

3. Breathe into the position, hold, and then slowly come up.

Note: If you are beyond the second trimester of pregnancy and/or are having trouble with your balance, try the Wall Squat instead of this pose.

35. Wall Squat

Benefits: The Wall Squat is a derivative of Malasana, only against the wall. Good for opening the pelvic area and stretching.

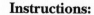

Instructions:

1. Get a blanket and place it facing the wall, not against it.

2. Lie on your back with your buttocks close to the wall and your legs vertical, up against the wall.

3. Separate your feet widely, placing the soles flat against the wall.

4. Put your hands on your knees and gently open the knees down with your hands. Do not force this movement.

5. Press your feet into the wall and breathe.

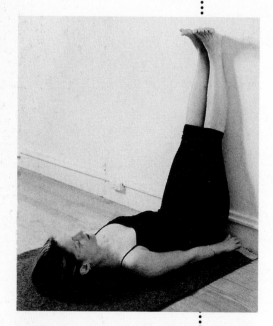

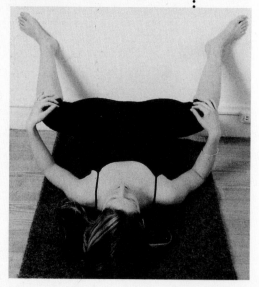

Surya Namaskara (The Sun Salutation)

Surya Namaskara, the Sun Salutation, is a pose that involves a sequence of twelve separate, flowing movements. Although it is taught as one of the basic postures, the Sun Salutation is not as easy as it looks. It should be taught by an instructor, as it contains backward, forward, and inverted positions.

Surya Namaskara is the prayer pose and a good warm-up. It is a prayer to the sun. *Surya* is "sun," and *namaskara* is "to bow." In the Sun Salutation, you literally bow gratefully to the sun. (Of course, it's nice if you can face the sun, but obviously that doesn't always happen.) The Sun Salutation is a wonderful exercise to greet the day, but make sure your body is warmed up. The body is not supple upon rising. You may need to take a warm shower to warm up your body. Some people use the practice of Surya Namaskara as their daily warm-up; others prefer to stretch before doing Surya Namaskara. Numerous poses in yoga evolve from the Sun Salutation. Surya Namaskara has something for the entire body, and many yogi masters postulate that if you do only one posture in your yoga practice, it should be the Sun Salutation. It limbers, stretches, and benefits the entire body.

Note: If you suffer from high blood pressure, are pregnant, or have eye problems, seek medical advice before starting the Sun Salutation.

Surya Namaskara begins in the same position as Tadasana.

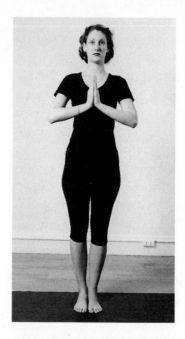

1. Bring your hands to your chest in a prayer position. Exhale.

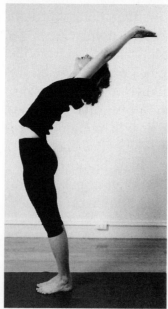

2. As you inhale bring your hands up over your head, keeping them close together and slightly tilting or arching the arms and head back. Hold.

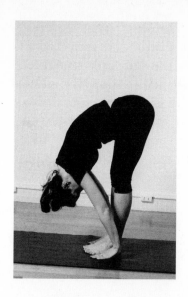

3. As you exhale stretch the arms forward, bending at the waist. Continue to slowly bend forward as far as you can go. (Go only as far as you can bend; do not push or bounce.) Ideally, the hands will touch the floor. Hold

4. Exhaling, extend your left leg back with your left knee touching the floor. Your right foot should still be on the floor and your right knee should be bent. Your hands are firmly on the floor parallel with the right foot. Lengthen your upper body upward. Look up, lifting your chin. Inhale in this position. Hold.

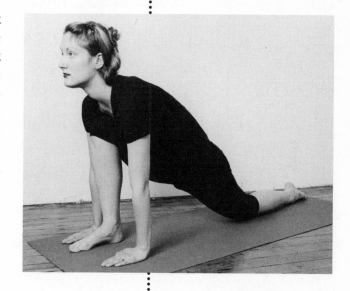

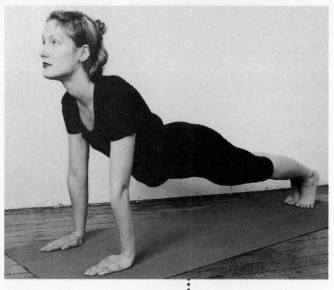

5. Holding your breath, bring your right foot back to join the left, and straighten both legs. Your shoulders should stay over your wrists. Your arms should be vertical and your toes tucked under, with the trunk of your body slightly off the floor.

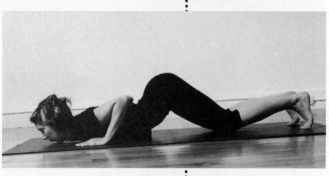

6. Exhaling, bend both your knees and elbows so that your toes and chest will touch the floor. Your rear will be slightly pushed into the air.

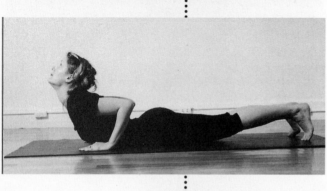

7. Inhaling, lower your body to the floor, keeping your arms at your sides, elbows bent. As your chest touches the floor, slowly lift your head back, and arch your upper back slightly. You are sustained by your hands and bent elbows. Don't straighten your arms or stress your spine. Hold.

8. Exhaling, use your arms and feet to arch your body up into a stretch. With the arms and legs straightened, your hands and feet stay on the floor. You are in an inverted V pose. Stretch and hold.

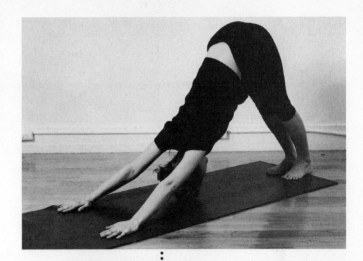

9. From the V, bring your left leg forward and put the heel on the ground as if kneeling. Extend the right leg all the way back, keeping the knee and toes on the ground. (The right leg should be stretched back, with the top of your foot on the floor, toes stretched out.) Inhale as your hips drop and the body lengthens.

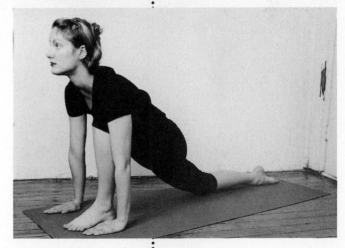

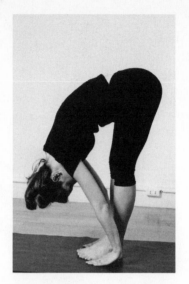

10. Exhaling, bring your back leg up to the left, and straighten your legs, keeping your body bent toward your knees and your hands on the floor. Hold.

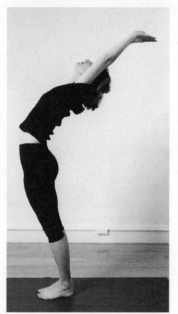

11. Inhaling, slowly extend your arms forward and up. Bending at the waist and keeping your hands close together, slightly arch your head and arms back as you did in step 2.

12. Exhale and bring your hands back to the prayer position, then down to your sides, standing in Tadasana—just as you began the Salutation in step 1.

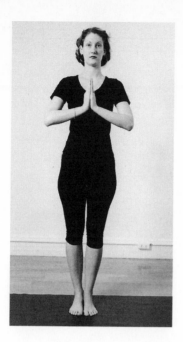

Learning about the asana may have enticed you to sign up for the first yoga class you find. But if you are new to yoga, you probably have some questions about classes and practicing on your own. Review chapter 5, "Finding a Class and Developing Your Yoga Practice," before you embark on a series of asana.

THE BOTTOM LINE

With hatha yoga, it is essential that you learn the asana correctly. There are numerous poses and variations to fit every need imaginable. Beginners should start slowly and work into more advanced poses. All asana afford a wealth of benefits for the individual, no matter what level of yoga one practices. You may find that your yoga teacher uses a different name or alters the poses slightly from this chapter. Regardless of style or variations, the benefits remain the same. The Sun Salutation is the root from which many of the postures sprouted. If you can't squeeze time into your routine for an extensive daily practice, make an effort to at least do the Sun Salutation: it alone will tone and stretch the entire body.

....

CHAPTER 5

Finding a Class and Developing Your Yoga Practice

THE KEYS

• Assess what you hope to gain from a yoga practice before beginning a class.

• There are some specific sources and tips to help you find a yoga teacher and a class.

• You won't need much to begin a yoga class, but you'll want to adhere to a few practical rules.

• Before practicing yoga at home, go through a checklist of obstacles that might impede a good practice.

• There are a number of yoga accoutrements to make your yoga practice easier.

Far too common is the yoga student who attends yoga classes beyond his or her level. Some recognize this immediately, and they search for a class that is better suited for them, or they talk to their instructor. Others follow diligently along without question. They are never quite sure if the asana they are doing are correct. Yet, they decline to ask questions or seek a level of yoga that may be a better match. What you learn in yoga class sets the foundation for your home practice. This chapter is a guide to finding a yoga class and developing a practice that suits your own personal needs.

Where to Begin: A Bit of Self-Assessment

In order to get the most from your yoga class, decide what you want from it. This will help you to determine what style of yoga to pursue. Are you taking a yoga class out of curiosity and because yoga has become so popular and you heard it was good for you? Or do you have a specific reason for taking yoga? Do you want to relax, learn to meditate, or get a good workout while stretching at the same time? As you know, the various types of yoga offer different approaches. What approach will work for your objectives?

Know Your Purpose

What has drawn you to yoga? What do you hope to obtain from yoga? Is taking a yoga class your idea or someone else's? These are some of the questions you might ponder before signing up for a class. Here are just a few common reasons people embark on a yoga class, some of which may be your own.

- To get in better physical shape

- For relaxation

- For mental and physical flexibility

- To strengthen the body

- For stress reduction

- Because a doctor recommended it

- Because I tried it at a spa and loved it

- For chronic pain

- For a disease

- To have fun

- To enhance spiritual direction

- Because it's popular

Keep in mind that your purpose for taking a class may change. If you begin a yoga class with the specific goal of learning to relax, and you do learn to do so, then your purpose for continuing yoga will change.

By defining concrete goals or what you hope to gain from a yoga practice, your expectations will be better met. If after taking a few sessions it is clear

STREET SMARTS

Joyce Thorton was dedicated to aerobics and worked out several times a week at the gym. "Some of the women in my aerobics class were doing yoga and kept touting the marvels of yoga. I felt pretty good with aerobics and didn't think yoga would enhance that feeling or make me feel better. Instead, I found the classes to be incredibly meditative and my body is certainly more flexible. I'm in tune with my body in a way that I wasn't with aerobics. Unfortunately, I'm not very disciplined about doing yoga at home, so I attend classes pretty faithfully. Yoga is now an integrated corner of my life. I teach preschool, and begin each class with the Sun Salutation. The students enjoy it and so do I."

that your expectations are different from those held by most others in your class, you should be willing to discuss your expectations with your yoga teacher. Express your expectations, so your yoga teacher can work with some of your needs in class.

Do You Have Special Concerns?

If you have a sports injury, back pain, chronic pain, or have special health concerns, you might consider a more therapeutic or meditative yoga class in lieu of a more physical yoga class.

Maybe you don't exercise regularly or are not in good physical shape but still want to take yoga. Start with a very gentle, beginning class. If you are currently under a physician's care, have high blood pressure or arthritis, or recently had surgery, check with your doctor before embarking on a yoga routine. Always let your yoga instructor know if you have a health problem or a health concern.

How Important to You Is the Yoga Environment?

It's no secret that environment is key to continuing success and attainment of goals when people undertake a new practice, endeavor to learn something new, or attempt to change their lifestyle. It's important that you self-assess the type of environment and the surroundings that you'll be comfortable in when you think about finding a class. This is just another way to ensure that you'll meet your objectives for pursuing yoga. Know what environment works best for you. Ask yourself these questions before you begin your search:

1. Are you easily distracted and do you find it difficult to focus in large groups? Do you feel you need absolute quiet to practice yoga or are you not bothered by occasional distractions?

2. Are you more comfortable in a small informal class or in a large class setting? Would you feel comfortable taking yoga in someone's home, at the local YMCA, or in a gym?

3. Will a photo of a guru, flowers, or the presence of incense or candles bother you?

4. Are you looking for a special style of yoga or a blend of styles? Does the location satisfy these needs?

5. Is the location convenient? Will this be an issue and a possible obstacle?

After you decide the purpose, the style, and the environment, it's time to search for a class and a teacher. Word of mouth or asking a friend who takes yoga is one way to find a teacher. (Remember, though, the style of yoga that you are looking for may not match your friend's style.) Another approach is to ferret out information on some of the styles you are interested in and sample a few different classes for at least a month and see what appeals to you. This is especially advisable if you are unclear about your purpose or what environment best suits you.

STREET SMARTS

Joel Sachs, a systems specialist from Annapolis, Maryland, speaks from experience when it comes to needing a yoga instructor: "I have taken yoga twice in my life, once to stretch my body for competitive rowing, the second time during a divorce when I needed some grounding. As far as I was concerned, yoga was yoga—no brand names or different styles. The first class was great. I felt like I was melting into the universe. It helped me let go, but I couldn't remember the sequence of poses once I got home. The biggest obstacle, though, was traveling all the time and the lack of discipline to practice on my own. I absolutely need a coach or teacher."

SMART MOVE

Julie Rappaport has been a yoga teacher for several years. She studied viniyoga in India and currently teaches viniyoga and prenatal yoga. "I can't stress how important it is to find a teacher who has studied or understands the traditions of yoga and the physiology of yoga. How your body and mind feel during a yoga class is important, but so is the relationship between the teacher and student. It should be one of comfort, sensitivity, and trust. It doesn't matter what kind of certification or experience a yoga teacher has; if you cannot connect with the teacher's method of teaching or if you feel uncomfortable in a class, it's best to look for another teacher or class."

Finding a Teacher

The most effective way to learn yoga is with a good teacher. This is not to say that you can't learn yoga on your own. However, only a teacher can observe you and make corrections; she or he can tell you if you are doing the asana and breathing correctly. In addition, if you have questions about how to get into the asana or if you feel some discomfort, the teacher can help you.

The Yoga Teacher Checklist

There is currently no required certification for teaching yoga nor is there an organization monitoring the quality and authenticity of yoga teachers. Anyone who wants to can invent a new brand of yoga and market it as a new lineage. Teachers' training programs vary and can range from a weekend to two years.

Several schools of yoga have strict certification programs, and there is a process underway to set up some type of certification for yoga teachers. Many teachers have a certification and have gone through a comprehensive accredited program. Others are not certified but have taught yoga for many years. As with any certification program, a yoga certification denotes that the individual has studied and obtained a certification at a particular school of yoga. On the other hand, many good yoga teachers are not certified, but have extensive or inclusive training.

You certainly want to make sure that the instructor you choose is knowledgeable and understands how to teach yoga. But, the most important component of finding a teacher is how you feel with that teacher, not whether he or she has a credential or has taught yoga for twenty years. As in any type of certification or program, it's the ability of the teacher to transmit his or her knowledge in a way that is appropriate and comfortable for you, the student, that matters.

When searching for a teacher, make a list of what you desire in a yoga teacher. The following are some prudent questions and considerations when considering a teacher.

• What is the teachers' training or experience?

• What types of yoga have they practiced or taught?

• How long have they been teaching?

• If you have an injury, such as a back problem, ask if the teacher has been trained to teach yoga for this specific injury. If not, ask them if they can suggest someone who has.

• What's the teacher's philosophy and methodology? Observe a class to make sure they match your own.

• Talk to the teacher and get an intuitive feeling for that individual.

• If you have inhibitions or concerns about the class, talk to the teacher more at length.

What Is a "Good" Yoga Teacher?

The American Association of Yoga defines a good yoga teacher as someone who:

• Has studied and comprehends the various effects of yoga exercises, breathing, and meditation.

• Is knowledgeable about the body's physiology.

• Is able to adapt techniques for each individual's capability.

• Adheres to yoga techniques and does not confuse religious or personal beliefs with yoga.

SMART SOURCES

Yoga Journal
2054 University
   Avenue, Suite 600
Berkeley, CA 94704
(800) I-DO-YOGA
Fax (510) 644-3101
The September issue
runs a special direc-
tory of yoga teachers.

Yoga International
Rural Route 1, Box
   407
Honesdale, PA 18431
(570) 253-4929

The American Yoga
   Association
513 South Orange
   Avenue
Sarasota, FL 34236
(941) 953-5859

The Yoga Finder is a
web page to help
locate classes and
teachers in the United
States:
www.chesco.com/
   yogafinder

Resources for Finding a Teacher

Check the yellow pages for yoga instructors or your local YMCA. Bulletin boards in health food stores, universities, health clubs, and metaphysical book-stores are all good sources for finding information on yoga classes.

If you are in a small town, don't have access to some of the above sources, or can't find the style of yoga you are looking for, pick up *Yoga Journal* or *Yoga International.* Both magazines annually print an extensive directory of yoga teachers and types of yoga classes available around the country.

Preparing for Yoga Class

You've decided what you want out of yoga and have investigated your options. You've found a class and a teacher that you think will meet your needs. And you're psyched to jump right in. Whoa! A little prep work will go a long way. Here's some advice:

• Wear loose clothing. Sweatpants or loose cot-ton pants and a T-shirt are fine. Some people pre-fer to wear loose-fitting, baggy shorts or a leotard.

• Many yoga centers or gyms have towels or mats to put on the floor. If they don't, however, you will need to bring your own. Schools of yoga that use props will have the necessary equipment available.

• Try to eat two hours prior to your yoga class. It is hard to do yoga on a full stomach. Conversely, if you are hungry, you will not be able to concentrate. If you must eat close to the time of class, eat some yogurt, fruit, or something very light an hour before class. Eating heavily can cause you to feel bloated and uncomfortable, making the asana more difficult to practice.

• Avoid doing heavy exercise or an intense workout prior to yoga class.

Tips for the Yoga Student in Class

Foremost, know your body. The teacher will demonstrate the postures and explain the movements. Watch and assimilate as much as you can. Be curious and don't be afraid to ask questions in class. Yoga is like anything else that you try; the more persistent and consistent you are with your yoga classes, the more you will benefit. Ask if you are doing a posture correctly. Ask for clarification if you are unsure of the breathing technique.

If you are unfamiliar with relaxation techniques or meditation, questions may arise around these subjects. By all means, ask them. Too often, it appears that everyone in class relaxes and meditates without a glitch, except you. Your mind is occupied with what to prepare for dinner or with the movie you want to see. Is this normal? Share your experiences; you might be surprised to find that others have the same worries.

Always ask the teacher to clarify what you may

not understand. Few of us go through life standing on our heads or sitting in a lotus position. So the first time you stand on your head or find your knees hurting from sitting cross-legged in your yoga class, questions will obviously arise. Ask them.

The following suggestions will both facilitate and maximize the benefits of your yoga class.

• **Be on time, if not early.** Yoga classes may last anywhere from sixty to ninety minutes. If you are continually late for class, you not only miss the beginning relaxation or asana but it shows a lack of respect for your teacher. It's best to arrive about ten or fifteen minutes early to get yourself into a relaxed state of mind. This is particularly important if you are taking class right after work, if you have a stressful day, or if you feel emotionally scattered.

• **Be attentive and focused.** Plan to stay through the entire class. Sometimes students are only interested in the asana, not the meditation or deep relaxation at the end of a class. If you commit to a yoga class, make the commitment to stay through the entire class. If you know you must leave early or arrive late, advise your teacher in advance.

• **Don't compare yourself to other yoga students.** Yoga is personal. Practice at your own pace. There will be many levels of students within a level of a yoga class. Some students move through the asana at a quicker pace or are able to hold the asana longer and with ease. Other students may be stiffer and take longer to get into an asana and quicker to come out of an asana. Stay focused and concentrate on what you can do.

• **Set reasonable, personal goals.** Do what you can and work at your own pace. Doing yoga should not be stressful; it is not the same as putting on your jogging shoes and taking a quick jog.

• **Be appreciative of corrections given by your teacher in class.** Accept posture, alignment, and breathing corrections and advice from your instructor, and do not regard these as criticisms.

• **Be patient with yourself and your practice.** Try not to become frustrated or give up at the first sign of difficulty or discomfort when you begin an asana or begin to meditate. Daily practice eases this discomfort.

• **Remember the quality of gratitude.** The relationship between the students and teacher in yoga is special and it always has been. In keeping with this tradition, it is always a nice gesture to thank your teacher. Sometimes your teacher may conclude a class by clasping her palms together bringing her hands to her heart as an expression of gratitude for the class. This movement may be followed by the word *namaste*. *Namaste* loosely translates as an expression of thank you to the class.

Assessing Your Class

The litmus test for how valuable your class is for you is how you feel when you take the class. You should feel relaxed, content, and restful. Your body should feel a tiny bit challenged, but not exhausted. You should not feel pain, and if you do,

F.Y.I.

Yoga teachers' training courses vary. Some are short, intense training courses, others span over a couple of years. Most follow a specific master's style of yoga. In a teacher's training, one should expect to study the yoga sutras, yoga philosophy, anatomy, asana, physiology, pranayama, and meditation.

your teacher should be open to discussing or acknowledging any problems.

If you feel agitated, defensive, or distracted, unfortunately, you've probably chosen the wrong teacher or class. But don't be discouraged, and don't throw the baby out with the bathwater: You know why you undertook yoga and are sure that it will address your needs. Consider looking for another class before deciding that yoga is not for you.

Your Personal Practice

You may find yourself inspired by a yoga class and excited to get home and practice the poses, only to find yourself standing in the middle of your living room wondering what to do or in what sequence to practice the asana.

This is not uncommon for beginners. Many people practice yoga at home, either on their own or in conjunction with taking classes. Setting up your own practice at home allows you to work at your own pace. You can concentrate on areas of your body that may be problematic, such as your back or hamstrings. You will also find that a home yoga practice will start to discipline and focus your daily activities. Nevertheless, it takes a little time to assimilate what you have learned in class in order to develop your own practice. Start slowly, and set goals.

Many people take a yoga class once a week for several months and then practice yoga on their own at home. Others take classes intensely, stop, practice at home, and begin more advanced classes when they are ready to learn more yoga.

Some thrive on classes, while others find the daily practice in their living room enough to meet their needs. Again, you'll need to assess what is best for your lifestyle.

Why Practice If You Are Taking a Class?

We live in times where most of us have more stress than relaxation in our lives. We expend energy in numerous directions; we are task oriented, have family obligations, get married, have a child, get divorced, and work when we should be sleeping. Our bodies respond to such stress, and we begin to operate reflexively, not mindfully. Sometimes resentment arises and other times we simply get sick. Taking the time to practice yoga allows you to get back in touch with your core self, helps to quiet the emotional layers of stress, and silences an overactive mind. The result is more harmony in your life. Doing a little bit of yoga in the morning is a wonderful way to start a day, just as practicing a bit in the evening can be a very restful way to conclude the day.

Obstacles to Your Routine

It is easy to sabotage a daily yoga practice. Time constraints and not enough hours in the day can impede the best of intentions. If obstacles continue to block your practice, you might ask yourself if you really want to practice yoga at home. If you do, then make a list of some of the obstacles that prevent you from practicing. According to an

STREET SMARTS

Charlie Salinger's purpose for beginning yoga was to increase his range of flexibility and range of motions. "A friend recommended yoga. I didn't have time for classes, and I preferred something I could do on my own. I picked up Richard Hittleman's *Yoga 28-Day Exercise Plan* and had a sense that it was a good program. The directions were simple and to the point. Within a month I noted improvement in my flexibility and I lost some weight. I often recommend yoga to my patients who are looking for more flexibility or range of motion in their joints and back or who have chronic back pain."

ancient yoga text, the most common obstacles to a yoga practice are lack of interest, doubt, laziness, false knowledge, failure to concentrate, pain, despair or depression, unsteadiness of the body, sickness, and unsteadiness of respiration.

Of these obstacles, only four have to do with the physical body. The rest are psychological. Be realistic with what you can accomplish at home, and do just that. Sure, it's nice to have an hour to practice yoga, but if you only have twenty minutes, then twenty minutes is better than nothing. It's better to practice yoga a little every day, or three or four times a week, than to do a weekend warrior stint of yoga on Saturday.

What You'll Need to Practice Away from Class

Foremost, you will need a quiet place to practice. Unplug the phone or mute your answering machine. Put your beepers to sleep. Turn off the television, radio, and computer. If you can't find a quiet corner in the house but you have a garden, you may want to practice outside. Some people go to a park or public garden.

If you have a family or little ones, find a time when you will not be disturbed. You may have to get up forty-five minutes earlier, wait until the family is asleep, or steal time in the afternoon to practice.

Set a precise time to practice and try to practice at the same time every day. This helps you stick to your daily practice even when you don't feel like

How to Transform Your House or Hotel into a Yoga Palace

When traveling and away from the place where you usually practice yoga, or even when practicing at home on your own, try to re-create an aesthetic or sacred practice space. Here are some tips:

- If the room has windows, let light in.

- Practice by candlelight.

- Set out a vase or drinking glass with a flower or flowers.

- If the room is bare bones, set out a small but peaceful photo, drawing, or postcard of something meaningful to you.

- If there is no mat to practice on, roll out a plush towel.

- Use a sofa or chair cushion for a bolster.

- If noise is a factor, put on a cassette or a CD with some calming, but never distracting, music.

doing it. And there will always be days you don't feel like doing yoga. These are the days to begin with your favorite poses and repeat them a few times. Be aware that some poses are stimulating and others more restorative. The poses you do will affect your mood and energy throughout the day. Don't do a stimulating series of poses before going to bed; and likewise, you may not want to start your day with restorative poses.

Begin with a short practice of about fifteen to twenty minutes and work up to thirty or forty-five minutes. If the longer time frame is not possible, but you really want to practice more, try two shorter sessions. If you can't squeeze breathing practices into your morning, try the three-part breathing practice while driving your car or on the bus or train. You might consider incorporating some simple stretching postures into your day, or you may start the day with a few asana and end the day with a deep relaxation. Be flexible. Yoga is not a militant practice.

In Practice, Bear in Mind . . .

When doing an activity away from a class or when alone and not in a group, it can sometimes be easy to lose focus and to slip up and be sloppy in your execution. Here are just a few reminders that will help you get the most out of your private yoga sessions. Remember:

• Keep in mind placement and body alignment. Consciously begin each pose and move slowly into each pose. Relax and go only as far as is comfortable in the poses. Listen to your body and don't overdo it.

• Don't become frustrated if you can't remember a pose; you can always consult a book or ask your teacher.

• Lengthen your stretch, but don't bounce in or out of poses.

• Breathe and remember to focus on your breath.

• Turn your attention inward, but avoid tensing muscles, including facial muscles.

• If you are in pain or if your body is tight, come out of a pose and trust your body. It's not your body that pushes you to pain, it is your ego egging you past your endurance.

• Practicing yoga at home should be enjoyable and relaxing. Don't practice when you are sick.

• If you use props, such as blankets or pillows, make sure you have them available so that you don't spend your time looking for them.

Spicing Up Your Practice Sessions

Like anything else you do repeatedly, you may become bored with your yoga routine. Change it! Start by changing the sequence of your poses or add some new ones. Try a few new or advanced poses. If you have a friend or family member who practices yoga, set a time to practice together.

Maybe it is time to enroll in a new yoga class or find a new yoga teacher. Keep in mind that even those who have practiced yoga for years have limitations that they must overcome.

Yoga Accoutrements

As yoga's popularity has soared, so has the commercialism of yoga, particularly in America. This is not to say that everyone who does yoga has yoga posters plastered across their walls or wears yoga T-shirts to class. Most people who do yoga do not have a commercial investment in it.

You can't *buy* the tradition of yoga, its health

SMART SOURCES

If you really want to spice up a practice, you may want to try and combine a yoga retreat with your interests or travel. There are hundreds of possibilities; many can be found in *Yoga Journal* magazine. Here are just a few:

Eco-Resort and Retreat Rancho Encantado, Mexico (800) 505-MAYA

Mana Le'a Gardens, Hawaii (800) 233-6467 with Rodney Yee

Pathways of Personal Growth Mount Madonna Center, California (408) 847-0406

Feathered Pipe Ranch, Montana (406) 442-8196

WHAT MATTERS, WHAT DOESN'T

What Matters

• That you find a teacher you like.

• That you have some personal yoga goals.

• That you respect your yoga teacher.

• That you feel comfortable talking with your yoga teacher.

• That you practice yoga at home with minimal interruptions.

What Doesn't

• Whether you travel a lot—yoga is portable and can be practiced wherever you are.

• The number or intensity of classes you take. If you take one class a week, you can still enhance your development by doing exercises and practicing breathing at home.

• That you don't want to attend yoga retreats.

• That you opt not to practice yoga at home.

benefits, or its spiritual component. These have no price tag and are not for sale. Nevertheless, there are yoga T-shirts, calendars, pranayama pillows, body and soul seminars, yoga magnets, physio balls, images, and charms—to mention a mere few, all for sale. There is nothing wrong with purchasing any items related to yoga. Some are inspirational, others merely decorative, and others give us a sense of well-being. You may be inclined to purchase some of these accoutrements, which is fine.

Remember though, yoga is a practice, and *you do not need to purchase anything to practice yoga.* Accoutrements will not make you a better yogi or yogini. Before the advent of sticky mats and meditation pillows, people tossed a towel or blanket on the floor, folded a feather pillow to sit on, and did yoga, and many still use these ordinary props.

The Props

When thumbing through yoga magazines or books, you'll notice people doing yoga with some interesting-looking contraptions—cotton straps, blocks, crescent-shaped pillows, or round, hard pillows. These are called props. If you're a novice yoga student or have taken a yoga class that does not use props, the idea of props may seem strange or it may pique your curiosity. Not everyone uses props for yoga, but many people do, and some find them most helpful.

The following is a list of some of the most common props and what they are used for. Some of these props are self-explanatory and others require some explanation. It's best to take a class or have an instructor show you how to use the props for alignment.

• **Yoga mats.** These are extremely light mats made from rubber and ranging in thickness. They are sometimes called sticky mats or traction mats. One side of the mat is sticky and adheres to the floor so that you don't slide. The mats come in colors, such as purple, blue, or gray, and range from $22 to $26 for thin mats. There are deluxe mats that are thicker and more expensive. Prices vary accordingly. Look for a mat that you can toss in the washer and roll up and put in a corner.

• **Blankets.** The blankets usually measure 50 × 80 inches or 60 × 80 inches, and are made of a firm or woven cotton or wool. The blankets are used in many poses for support of the head, back, neck, legs, and other areas.

• **Bolsters.** Bolsters are round or rectangular cushions that are cotton filled. Round bolsters are approximately 26 inches long by 9 inches in diameter; rectangular bolsters measure 7 × 12 × 25 inches. They are used in numerous ways to support your body and help attain various postures. Rolled towels or small chair cushions will work, as well.

• **Blocks.** Lightweight wood or foam blocks are approximately 4 × 6 × 9 inches, and are used under your feet or hands to help you get into a pose.

• **Cotton straps with D-ring buckles.** These straps are available in standard lengths of 6 and 9 feet, and are used for stretching in poses.

• **Sandbags.** These 5- and 10-pound sand-filled bags (which can also easily be made) are used in postures for support or to attain a pose.

SMART SOURCES

Good sources for everything you could (materially) need to do yoga:

Bheka Yoga Supplies
(800) 366-4541
www.yogavoices.com.
   bheka

Fish Crane
P.O. Box 791029
New Orleans, LA
   70179
(800) 959-6116

Yogamats
P.O. Box 885044
San Francisco, CA
   94118
(800) 720-YOGA
[800-720-9642]

THE BOTTOM LINE

Learning to do yoga correctly is vital. The first order of the day is to find a good teacher and yoga class. To do this, shop around—ask questions and talk to people. Some teachers are certified and some are not. The most important aspect of a teacher is how you feel about that teacher's ability to teach you yoga. Once you find a yoga class, be attentive and arrive on time. You might want to practice yoga at home; if so, find a quiet place and a regular time of day to practice. If the style of yoga you are doing requires props, learn how to use them and have them handy. Ultimately, yoga is just like any other practice that requires some dedication; it can have obstacles. Evaluate them to overcome them.

• **Zafus.** These are hard round or crescent-shaped pillows used for meditation. They are more comfortable than sitting on a flat floor.

• **Benches.** Small lightweight wooden benches are sometimes used instead of the floor or a pillow for sitting during meditation by individuals who find sitting on a floor or pillow difficult.

Now that you have found a great yoga teacher and the right class, a perfect place at home to practice, and are at ease practicing the asana, the next step is learning to meditate. But before we journey into meditation, let's glance at the body's chakras, in chapter 6.

....

The Body's Chakras

Chakras are psychic centers of activity, or of the vital force of prana, that cannot be defined in terms of psychology, physiology, or any other science. Chakras are interrelated with the parasympathetic, sympathetic, and autonomous nervous systems. In this chapter we discuss the aspects of the chakras.

What Is a Chakra?

Chakra is the Sanskrit word for "wheel." The wheels are rotating energy centers within the body, and they are always active. If you are acquainted with physics or quantum physics, in which movement occurs continuously at the atomic particle level, the continual movement within the chakras will not be a difficult concept to grasp.

Each chakra is connected to an emotional and psychological function within the astral or emotional body and physical body. Because the human body is in a constant state of flux, human behavior influences the chakras.

Western and Eastern Approaches

When we begin talking about universal energy or energy channels, a subject that cannot be quantified or verified, we may question its existence. In yogic and Eastern thought, what is essential is not always visible to the eye. Chakras are an essential component of the yogic anatomy. Nevertheless, they are invisible and are not taught in human anatomy in the West. For most of us, the mention of the visible or tangible is pretty easy to digest, but the idea of working in the invisible or intangible realm drums up doubts or conflicting notions.

In order to understand the significance of chakras, we must look at the way both Eastern and Western medicine approach the body and the mind. There is a sea of differences between the way the West approaches medical philosophy and the way the East approaches it.

Western Medical Philosophy

Western medicine is based on the Cartesian philosophy; that is, the body represents one functioning system and the mind another. The mind and body are two separate entities. In Western medicine, the emphasis is on a rational approach. Western science works in the realm of proven truths; if it can't be proven, it probably isn't true.

Some doctors, however, are beginning to challenge this approach. Recent medical research has begun to uncover scientific truth behind the mind-body connection.

Eastern Medical Philosophy

In Eastern medicine, the approach to the physical body and the mind is more connective. The mind and the body are not looked upon as separate entities, but merge holistically as one intimate entity. Eastern medicine acknowledges that if something is stressing the mind, it will provoke symptoms in

SMART SOURCES

In 1988, Herbert Benson, M.D., professor of Medicine at Harvard Medical School, founded the Mind/Body Institute in Deaconess, Massachusetts, outside of Boston. The institute is affiliated with six hospitals nationwide and when established was a radical departure from traditional care. In 1995 Benson established the Center for Training in Mind/Body Medicine in Boston, which teaches clinicians how to practice mind/body medicine.

Mind/Body Medical
 Institute
110 Francis St.
 Suite 1A
Boston, MA 02215
(617) 632-9530
www.mindbody.harvard.
 edu

the body, and vice versa. It postulates that health is achieved and disease prevented by maintaining the body in a balanced state, thus physical and mental well-being must be combined. In Ayurvedic medicine, the Indian science of life and longevity, the body's energy unit needs to be in balance in order to hum along in a healthy state. Naturopathic doctors in India subscribe to a similar outlook regarding the body and mind. When the chakras become blocked, both the mind and the body can experience pain, stress, or discontentment.

Chakra Points

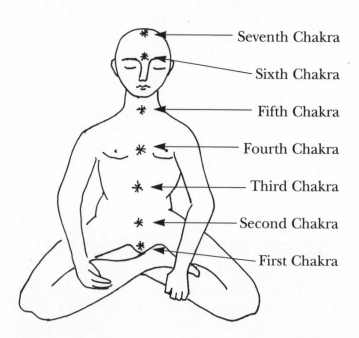

Seventh Chakra

Sixth Chakra

Fifth Chakra

Fourth Chakra

Third Chakra

Second Chakra

First Chakra

Drawing by Nadine Gay

The chakras absorb prana and distribute it through the channels, or nadis, to the nervous system, the endocrine system, and the blood. The act of fine-tuning or unclogging the energy channels in the body results in greater well-being.

There are seven major chakra points and twenty-one minor chakra points. The minor points are distributed throughout the body, and the seven majors are located along the spine, from the base to the crown of the head. The major chakras work with the endocrine glands in the physical body. Prana flows through the chakras. When a chakra is blocked, the corresponding endocrine gland performs poorly.

The Seven Major Chakras

Both yogic thought and Ayurvedic medicine recognize and accept the fact that the chakras rest within the astral body or emotional body. Chakras cannot be described in general psychological or physiological science as the empirical mind prefers. One cannot touch chakras or see them.

The chakras act as an interchange or liaison between our physical and psychological energy. This energy or prana, the life force, travels up the body. Through meditation, visualization, asana, and mantra techniques, the yogi strives to clear blocked energy in the chakra regions.

The seven major chakras have specific locations in the body, and each chakra corresponds to physical functions in the body. In esoteric Eastern thought, the chakras are symbolized by a color and an element. Each chakra is depicted by lotus petals

SMART SOURCES

For more information or referrals regarding Naturopathic doctors in your area, write to the following address:

The American Association of Naturopathic Physicians
2366 Eastlake Ave. E. Suite 322
Seattle, WA 98102

The Coils of Kundalini

Kundalini is derived from *kundala,* meaning a "ring" or "coil." This cosmic energy is symbolized as a sleeping serpent with three and a half coils. The three coils represent the three states of the mind:

1. *Jagrat,* awake

2. *Svapna,* dreaming

3. *Susupti,* deep sleep

The half coil represents the fourth state of the mind, *Turiya,* which is the transcendence of the other states, or the enlightened state.

Source: Light on Pranayama: The Yogic Art of Breathing, B. K. S. Iyengar

corresponding with the number of nadis, or nerve channels, emanating from each chakra. The chakras are referred to in ascending order beginning with the lowest or base chakra. This is where the kundalini is located. The kundalini, or dormant energy, is always represented by a coiled snake. In order for the energy to rise up through the chakras, the kundalini must uncoil.

The First Chakra

The first chakra is Muladhara. It translates as "root" and is symbolized as a deep red lotus flower with four petals. It is located at the base of the coccyx in the lower spine near the three lower vertebrae. This is our center of physical vitality and energy, and this chakra regulates our sense of smell. The endocrine glands associated with it are the gonads, the testes in the male and the ovaries in the female. Maladhara's element is earth, and it is concerned with our roots and source of security. This is called the foundation chakra and contains the primal energy or the kundalini.

The Second Chakra

The second chakra is Svadhisthana. It translates as "one's own abode or place of dwelling" and is depicted with six petals that radiate the color orange.

The second chakra sits below the navel near the pubis area. It is associated with the skin, the reproductive organs, the kidneys, the bladder, and the circulatory and lymphatic systems. Water is the element of the second chakra, and water is the essence of life. This chakra is linked with our emotions, fears, anxieties, and our sexuality.

The Third Chakra

The third chakra is Manipura, and it means "city of jewels." It is represented by ten bright yellow lotus petals. Manipura is located in the solar-plexus area of the body, below the heart. The element of the third chakra is fire, the provider of vital energy. This is the meeting point in which prana, the upward moving vital energy, and apana, a downward moving vital energy, link. Heat in the body is generated from this point. This is also the center of desire and emotion, ego and personal power. In the physical body, this is the spot where digestion and food absorption occur, which affect the stomach, duodenum, gall bladder, and liver. The endocrine gland associated with this chakra is the pancreas.

The Fourth Chakra

The fourth chakra is Anahata and it means "unstuck." It is depicted as a green lotus with twelve petals. It is physically associated with the heart and the circulatory, lymphatic, respiratory, and immune systems. The endocrine association is the thymus. This is the heart chakra, and it rests in the cardiac region or chest. The Anahata chakra is the center

SMART DEFINITION

The Lotus Flower

The lotus flower symbolizes our human spiritual evolution. The root in the soil represents our lowest nature. The stem, which develops from water, denotes our intuitive endeavors; and the flowering lotus blossom, which develops from the sun, represents self-realization.

of compassion. It is the balancing chakra between the lower and upper chakras. Here is where one experiences love or hate, compassion or emotional restriction. Love has many different natures. It can be restricted or demanding, or it can be passionate or unconditional. When one's heart is not open or is in pain, the body, mind, and spirit cannot attain balance. The element for Anahata is air.

The Fifth Chakra

The fifth chakra is Vishuddha and it means to "purify." Vishuddha is symbolized by a sixteen-petal smoky-violet blue lotus. This chakra is located in the throat and is associated with the sense of hearing. This is the chakra of knowledge, communication, and creativity. It is concerned with how one expresses oneself or how one communicates before the world. It governs our nervous system, vocal cords, and ears. The element of the fifth chakra is ether. The endocrine glands associated with it are the thyroid and parathyroid.

The Sixth Chakra

The sixth chakra is Ajna and it is depicted with two lotus petals in the center of the brow. It translates as "command." The petals represent reasoning and intuition, or the duality of our ego and our spiritual halves. It sits between the eyebrows and is sometimes called the "third eye," or the intuitive powers. Ajna is associated with the color indigo. This is the center of concentration for meditation. It correlates with increased memory, willpower, and visual-

Characteristics of the Seven Major Chakras

Each of the seven major chakras has a corresponding color, and each chakra represents specific emotions or qualities. Here's a simple chart of the chakras' characteristics.

Chakra	Color	Quality
First Chakra	Red	Security and roots
Second Chakra	Orange	Sexuality and emotions
Third Chakra	Yellow	Our sense of self
Fourth Chakra	Green	Love, devotion, compassion
Fifth Chakra	Blue	Communication, knowledge
Sixth Chakra	Indigo	Intuition
Seventh Chakra	Crystalline	Union with the divine, or self-realization

ization; and physically with the eyes, ears, nose, and brain. This is the sun chakra, the brilliance of a pure consciousness. When out of balance, confusion and irritability may dominate. The endocrine gland associated with Ajna is the pituitary. Before one can tap into intuitive powers, excess mental activity in this chakra must be cleared.

The Seventh Chakra

The seventh chakra is Sahasrara, or the chakra of supreme existence. It is located at the crown of the head and represents infinity. This is the center

Karen Ansaldo uses the chakra points in her massage practice. "I'm not a chakra expert, but I use the energy of each chakra as a map as to what is going on inside the person's body. I begin the massage by placing my hand over each chakra point. This allows me to connect with the individual's energy. The chakras act as a guide or circuit alerting me to what is blocked and what areas of the body need working on. Sometimes the chakras are stronger in one area and weaker in others."

of consciousness, called the "thousand-petaled" chakra. All feelings, activities, and emotions are calm and silent in this chakra. When the seventh chakra is unblocked, it represents the guru within each of us who is self-luminescent.

The Belief in Chakras and Yoga

Yoga does not have to involve working with the chakra. In fact, some yoga texts just skim over the chakras and a few don't even mention them at all.

Your yoga teacher most likely will not incorporate chakra exercises. Some systems of yoga do not work with the chakras, while others, such as tantra and kundalini yoga, work extensively with the chakra energy. Your teacher may incorporate the chakra points in a meditation or perhaps mention them. He or she might ask you to visualize or focus on a particular area of the body that is troubling you.

Chakra Clearing

Still a little skeptical about the subject of chakras but somewhat intrigued? Here's a chakra cleansing to connect the psychic body to the somatic body. This chakra cleansing exercise can be done in about fifteen minutes and is a nice way to end the day. It taps into the energy flow that runs through the entire body. It requires some visualization and gentle breathing, and preparation is minimal.

1. Sit comfortably in a quiet place. If you can cross your legs and sit in the Easy Pose, do so. Keep your spine straight. If you cannot sit cross-legged, modify the position; you can sit in a chair or lie on your back.

2. Relax and take a few deep breaths.

3. Close your eyes.

4. You are ready for the chakra-clearing visualization technique.

Chakra-Clearing Visualization Technique

1. Visualize a crystal clear stream of water entering the top of your head through the crown. Visualize it washing away all the stresses of the day.

2. As the stream flows down to the "third eye" it turns indigo. Visualize the cool stream of water washing away the day's mental anxiety.

3. The stream of water moves down the neck and into the throat, turning blue. The blue stream washes away all the things you wish you'd said or hadn't said during the day, all the miscommunication and bothersome nuances, clearing the way for good communication.

4. As the stream of water moves down into your chest, it turns a radiant healing green, circling the heart. Many of us hold fear in this area, and the green stream washes the fear away, making room for compassion.

WHAT MATTERS, WHAT DOESN'T

What Matters
• That you sit straight with the spine erect if you do a chakra cleansing.

• That you feel comfortable whether or not you decide to incorporate the chakras into your practice of yoga.

• That you don't get hung up on not being able to explain chakras to you family, friends, or doctor.

• That your practice yoga even if you don't believe in chakras.

What Doesn't
• Being able to see the chakras.

• Being able to feel the chakras.

• That Western medicine doesn't have scientific proof of chakras.

5. The stream descends to the solar plexus, turning a brilliant yellow. Visualize the yellow stream cleansing away doubts about your personal self, allowing you to freely express your true self.

6. As the stream is drawn downward into the belly or navel area, it turns orange. The orange stream cleanses all the anger or personal frustration about yourself, freeing penned-up energy.

7. As the stream enters the first chakra, it turns ruby red. Visualize the red stream cleansing what you have held on to, and let it wash away excess worldly weight. Taking a deep breath, let the red stream flow out through your toes.

8. Continue to inhale and exhale, and imagine all the colors converging and turning into a beautiful clear stream of water. The stream bubbles up through each chakra and out the top of your head, showering you with a fountain of clear energy.

Source: Adapted from *The Holistic Health Handbook,* compiled by Berkeley Holistic Health Center, 1978.

You may find the idea of chakras refreshingly enlightening or too esoteric and a bit obscure for your liking. In either case, remember this: Yoga—and the decision to study and/or incorporate chakras—is a matter of personal choice. So is the topic of the next chapter, meditation. Chapter 7 answers common questions about meditation and delves into a myriad of meditation methods for you to explore.

THE BOTTOM LINE

Chakras may be a new phenomenon for you, and that's okay. They are an ancient part of yogic and Ayurvedic thought. The body has seven chakras that run along the spine and correspond to endocrine functions in the body. Prana runs through the chakras and begins its ascent at the base of the spine, moving up through the navel and solar plexus, into the heart region, passing up into the throat, ascending into the "third eye" region, and exiting out the crown of our head. You may or may not encounter chakra exercises in your yoga class.

CHAPTER 7

Meditation and Yoga

THE KEYS

• Meditation is both a tool for personal growth and a powerful antidote for an overactive mind.

• There are several meditative techniques that one can use to open up to the practice. Some of the techniques will be new to you; others you may be familiar with.

• There are numerous hows, whens, and whys concerning effective meditation.

• The health benefits associated with meditation are numerous and undisputed in medical and scientific circles.

• Meditation can be done in a group or solo, and there are benefits to each method.

Meditation is not about feeling a particular way, or about getting somewhere psychologically, or about just relaxation. Meditation is the practice of stilling the mind. Although meditation is not a mainstream practice, physicians, researchers, and scientists have clearly established that meditation can play an important role in medical healing.

In major medical institutions across the country, meditation courses have been incorporated into stress-reduction programs, HMO health education programs, heart disease programs, and research studies. Nevertheless, the majority of Americans that meditate do so not for a particular medical problem but to go about deepening their quotidian awareness, to refine their attention, and for the sense of well-being associated with meditation practices.

What Is Meditation?

Meditation is discovery, the unfolding of the mind. While meditation is often considered an esoteric religious rite, it is actually a tool that aims to strengthen the mind's ability to sustain attention. Meditation is a sequential component of a yoga practice; part of a process. The first step is doing the asana, which helps ready the body for the second step—pranayama or breathing practices. Pranayama helps with concentration, and that sets the mood for meditation. The practice of asana and pranayama, yoked together, pave the way for the mind to focus and to meditate.

In meditation, the mind is not asleep but focused. Try and visualize the process of meditation as a bell curve. Foremost, at the flat part of the bell, you begin by eliminating the obstacles that prevent you from focusing. In yoga, the breathing techniques and asana help you here. You arrive at the crest or dome of the bell when your mind can remain focused. When you close or finish your meditation, you ultimately return your awareness to a normal state or level.

But what does meditation *actually* do, and why is it so important? Here are some of its *proven* benefits:

- It encourages relaxation.

- It increases awareness.

- It enhances mental clarity.

- It bathes the mind with a sense of peace.

Meditation and the Mind

Sitting still and quieting the mind takes perseverance and practice. Asking an adult to still or quiet the mind is comparable to asking a two-year-old to sit quietly and not wiggle—very difficult, indeed. The majority of us spend our days bombarded by sensory input. The mind is active—we engage it in reading, studying, writing, conversing, watching television, or spending hours in front of a computer screen. The mind seldom reposes or gets a wink of rest. Our bodies would revolt or get sick if

F.Y.I.

The Yoga Sutras list five possible states of mind:

1. Agitated. The mind that wanders everywhere, but ends up nowhere.

2. Distracted. The mind that tries to focus on an object but becomes easily distracted.

3. Dull. The mind is not totally present; it is lethargic.

4. Focused. The mind remains attentive and focused, although it has not attained perfect clarity.

5. Absorption. The evolved mind, or the state in which the mind has no distractions. Nothing hinders absorption in this state.

The mind generally hovers among the first three states. The last two states are when meditation can actually take place.

we pushed them to keep up an equivalent pace—for example, biking, running, and swimming all day with no warm-up or break—for too long. Mentally, however, during our waking hours our minds channel-surf, tossing from one activity to another. All this agitation disturbs concentration. Theoretically, during meditation all the mental activity settles down. The mind doesn't go to sleep, but meditation allows it to become peaceful, calm, and aware.

Two Techniques to Calm the Mind

In yoga, the metaphor for the mind is likened to a chattering monkey that has been bitten by a scorpion. Meditators use different techniques in order to hush all the static in the mind.

Meditation is not about zoning out. Quite the opposite; it requires the mind to focus its attention on one object or on a moment-to-moment awareness. There are traditionally two techniques used to meditate—*concentrative* and *mindfulness*. Some forms of meditation combine the techniques. Depending on the method of meditation, the focus of attention may vary. The goal, regardless of the method or object of focus, is to hush mental activity.

Concentrative Meditation Technique

This practice focuses on a concrete object, such as a candle, the breath, or a sound or mantra, on which the mind is able to dwell. If the mind meanders or drifts, the object or sound serves to refocus the attention.

Mindfulness Meditation Technique

This practice is a little more complicated. Instead of focusing on an object or sound, you acknowledge the feelings floating through your mind, but you do not engage the feelings or thoughts; you witness or observe them dispassionately and without judgment.

Helpful Hints to Prepare for Meditation

Breathing Meditation Exercise

Awareness of your posture is vital in a meditation practice. Sit in the Easy Pose (page 65) and relax the eyes. Close them, and concentrate on your inhalation and exhalation. Invariably, your attention will wander. Intruding thoughts will pop up while you're trying to concentrate on your breathing cycle. Don't squelch or fixate upon them. Gently bring your attention back to your breathing.

Foremost, understand your purpose for meditating. Is it medical or spiritual? Is it for stress reduction or to refine inner awareness? Is it because you want to meditate or because someone else told you it would be good for you? It is easier to practice meditation if you define or clarify your purpose for meditation.

Meditation is highly individual. The technique or techniques your teacher uses in a yoga class may not suit you. You may need to shop around for a technique that suits your lifestyle.

Certain meditation traditions from other cultures may not be harmonious with your culture or traditions. Meditation experiences differ significantly. While much has been written about the benefits of meditation, it's best not to have expectations. Meditation is about becoming aware and sensitive to what occurs within you. It is not an escape from reality, or a retreat into a cave. It is a practice that leads to harmony and reality. Meditation is an illumination of reality, not an escape from it.

Sitting for Meditation

As with all aspects of yoga, sitting for meditation requires proper positioning, form, and concentration, although these should be achieved in your own individual way. Here are some basics for preparing the sitting pose for meditation.

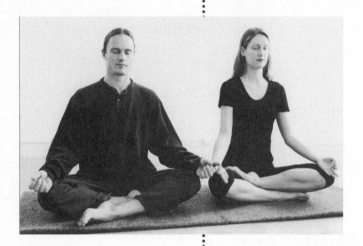

• Beginners may want to sit against a wall in the Easy Pose. Let your knees drop toward the floor. Take care with your knees in sitting meditation; do not compromise them by forcing them into a painful position. Let the knees drop only as far as they can naturally.

• Sit straight with your head and neck erect and your spine straight. Imagine an invisible string running through your spine which connects the crown of your head to the heavens and roots the base of your spine to the earth.

• Your weight, when sitting, should be distributed evenly on the buttocks.

• Ease your back forward to meet your chest.

• Adjust your position for comfort.

• If your feet begin to feel numb from being tucked under your legs, adjust their position.

• Make sure the room is conducive to relaxation and you are dressed comfortably and warmly.

• If you can't sit on the floor in this position, sit in a chair with your feet on the ground, spine erect, and your hands on your lap.

Meditation Styles

You may not be interested in meditation at all and decide to skip this chapter; or you may feel content with the brief meditation at the end of your yoga class. Certainly, you can practice yoga without practicing a formal meditation. Nevertheless, many individuals happen upon meditation in a class and quickly discover that meditation adds another dimension to their lives. Nuances of tranquillity appear; these people feel peaceful, sleep better, and

Walking Meditation Exercise

This exercise is one that combines meditation with motion. In a quiet, bucolic environment, mindfully begin to walk slowly and with intention. Connect your breathing with each footstep. Each step becomes a meditation. Although you physically move in this type of meditation, each movement is articulated and slow.

Fertile Seeds for Focusing the Mind

Before you settle down to the actual practice of meditation, try a few of the following exercises to focus the mind. They are good primers to concentrate the mind and prepare it for meditation.

Botanical Practice

Find a garden and focus on one flower. Notice its color, fragrance, and size. Reflect on the characteristics of the petals. Are they velvety, polished, delicate, scalloped, sensuous, or thorny? Then close your eyes and recall every detail of the flower.

Artistic Practice

The next time you are in an art gallery, stop in front of a painting that you especially like. Reflect on the color, style, brush strokes, and physical characteristics of the piece of art. Pay attention to sensations the painting evokes. Walk away from the painting and see what you remember about it. Repeat the exercise with a painting that you don't like.

Literary Practice

When reading a book, stop at the end of the page and see if you can recall what you read on that page. Can you recall how many paragraphs there were on the page, any quotes, or the title of the chapter?

Quotidian Practices

The next time you take a walk, focus on your breathing. Make breathing the focus of your walk. In the car, if you are a passenger or if you are stuck in traffic, shut off the radio and focus on the sounds and sights around you.

acquire another level of awareness. These are pleasing sensations that individuals want to intensify, and so they embark on a meditation practice.

There are numerous techniques for meditation. How one chooses to meditate is very personal. While you may want to experiment with a few different techniques, it's a good idea to find one meditation style that is compatible with you.

The following are some of the different ways that people practice meditation. Not all of the meditation practices are taught in yoga classes.

Transcendental Meditation

Transcendental Meditation, known as TM, is not taught in yoga classes. Scores of individuals who meditate and practice yoga today were introduced to meditation in the 1960s by Maharishi Mahesh Yogi. By the 1970s, more people were practicing TM than any other form of meditation.

Transcendental Meditation does not use asana or pranayama to prepare the mind for meditation; TM's sole focus is on meditation.

A trained instructor gives you a secret sound called a mantra. The sound or mantra resonates with the individual. After receiving the mantra from the teacher, the individual meditates twice a day for twenty minutes using the mantra. According to Joseph Vella, who is a certified yoga instructor and has been practicing TM since 1974, "In TM, you let your thoughts be, you don't observe or witness them and there is no object of focus. The repetition of the mantra becomes effortless, the sound seems to slip away, and meditation becomes automatic. I found TM to have an overwhelmingly positive effect on my thoughts and attitudes."

F.Y.I.

In 1968 practitioners of Transcendental Meditation came to Harvard Medical School and asked if they could participate in a study to show that meditating could lower blood pressure. Herbert Benson, M.D., the lead researcher, found that the participants in the study evoked a bodily response he called "the relaxation response," the opposite effect of the fight-or-flight response. Physiologically, Dr. Benson found that the body responds to meditation by:

• A decrease in blood pressure

• A decrease in heart rate

• A decrease in breathing rate

• A decrease in the metabolic rate

Source: The Relaxation Response, Herbert Benson, M.D.

SMART SOURCES

If you want to hear what a mantra can actually sound like, the musician Paul Horn recorded this sound in an album titled *Paul Horn Inside the Taj Mahal*.

Mantra, or Japa, Yoga

A *mantra* is a sacred Sanskrit sound or syllable from a word that has a particular vibration. *Japa* is the repetition of the mantra. Each mantra has a certain quality to it and has been chosen by a teacher or sage especially for the individual. Many people use mantras to meditate; however, not everyone has a specific mantra or has ever practiced Transcendental Meditation, which requires a mantra.

You don't need a teacher to give you a mantra; there are universal mantras that people use. There is no market on mantras. The most widely practiced mantra is "Om" or "Soham." Om is considered a universal vibration or sound that most anyone can use. Om is used in many yoga classes as is Soham, which means "I am that." When you chant these mantras, the sound should start deep in your throat, moving the vibration up through your head.

Mala Beads and Mantra Meditation

Another way to practice japa meditation is with the physical aid of mala beads. The string of 108 beads is held in the right hand. Each bead is rolled with the thumb and a finger, one by one, as you repeat and focus on your mantra.

Chanting

Another way of using a mantra is to chant it.

"Not chanting," you may protest, "it's bizarre, too weird to even contemplate. Besides, why chant when you don't know what you are chanting?"

This is a pretty common reaction when chanting comes up. The idea of chanting often turns many people off on meditation completely. People feel inhibited about chanting and are surprised by the effect chanting has on calming the mind and body once they try it. Much the way a hymn or spiritual song seems to move or elevate the mind to a joyous plateau, so does chanting. Chanting is about contacting the subconscious mind. Nevertheless, in keeping with the yoga philosophy of doing what is comfortable, chant only if you wish to.

Tratak

Tratak is a visual technique that helps focus concentration. It requires the eyes to be partially closed as they gaze upon one object intensely for a period of time. Try not to blink or take your eyes from the object. Then, close your eyes and visualize the object in your mind. One of the best ways to try tratak is by gazing at the flame of a candle for as long as you can. Place the candle at eye level in a darkened room. Stare at it for two or three minutes before closing your eyes. Once you close your eyes, you will be able to see the glow and shape of the candle in your mind. Some individuals use a flower or other object. Again, this is a matter of personal preference.

Symbols

Sometimes a person uses a symbol or photo of a spiritual object, a saint, or something sacred to meditate on. Others have small altars with a photo of a saint or guru, flowers, or a symbolic item that they use for meditation. Symbols are extremely personal. The advantage of a symbol is that it is able to transcend cultural barriers. What symbolizes something sacred to one individual may not

STREET SMARTS

Connie Mazzella discovered chanting through Integral Yoga teachers training. "Annually we had three-day silent retreats. At the end of each day we chanted. It was the best part of the day for me. The unity in the room energized me in a way I had never experienced. Chanting, or *kirtans,* is not about the voice or ability to carry a tune; it's about allowing your energy to flow. People are inhibited about chanting; no one really wants to open their mouth and belt out a chant. I led a monthly chanting group in San Francisco and encouraged the use of small instruments—little drums, bells, tambourines, maracas, which are typically used with chanting. People were as inhibited about picking up the instruments as they were about chanting. Once a few people grabbed an instrument, the rest of the group joined in. The energy in chanting is remarkable."

F.Y.I.

Frederic M. Luskin, Ph.D., at the Complementary and Alternative Medicine Program at Stanford School of Medicine (CAMPS), one of the ten National Institutes of Health research centers on alternative and complementary medicine, has documented the positive effects of meditation in curbing stress and anxiety for individuals with cardiovascular problems. A recent pilot study looked at another segment of the population: teachers. Teaching has one of the highest turnover rates of any profession due to stress. The study found that the meditation group significantly reduced their stress symptoms in the "domains of emotional manifestations, gastrointestinal distress and behavioral manifestations."

Source: "The Effect of a Meditation Program on the Level of Stress in Secondary School Student Teachers," Frederic M. Luskin, Ph.D., and Andrew J. Winzelberg, Ph.D.

have the same meaning to another. To many yogis, one of the most powerful symbols is that of the Sanskrit letters for "Om."

Mandala

A *mandala* is a circular design that draws the eye to the center of the circle. Mandalas are colorful and complex and take a variety of forms, from a simple geometric pattern to more elaborate, complicated patterns. Some mandalas are elaborate paintings on cloth. The mandala is profoundly symbolic in certain cultures. It is the foremost symbol allegorically in Tibetan Tantra Buddhism for man's relationship with the cosmos or the spiritual path of the body and mind. Outside of Grace Cathedral in San Francisco, there is a mandala. The famous cathedral at Chartres, France, has a mandala on its floor.

In meditation a mandala represents the path to enlightenment. When one meditates on the colors in the mandala, the visual stimulation awakens the mind, body, and spirit.

Mindfulness Meditation

This type of meditation grew out of Buddhist meditation practice, and it refers to the state of being awake or mindful. Mindfulness meditation means paying attention, in a particular way, to the present moment or situation. You don't change the moment or situation, you simply acknowledge it without judgment. Mindfulness meditation nurtures awareness.

Your Choice: Group or Solo?

Now that you have discovered all these wonderful techniques, how do you actually apply them? Should you meditate in a group setting or do it solo? Should you get up at dawn or meditate at night? And how much time can you possibly eke out to meditate with an already overcommitted schedule? Let's start with the actual sitting.

Group Sittings

For many, their first contact with meditation is in a yoga class with other people present. Other individuals, who do not practice yoga, participate in group meditation that specifically teaches one technique. Others find a group that teaches a variety of meditation techniques. Group meditations might gather once a week for a specific period of time to practice. A group's participants have the opportunity to share their experiences and feelings about meditation.

Solo Sittings

On the home front, meditation typically remains a private experience not shared with household members, unless, of course, they meditate. Individuals may carve out a corner in their home to meditate. If meditation is a new practice in your home, you may have to explain to your family or room-

SMART MOVE

Robert Stahl teaches an eight-week mindfulness program at El Camino Hospital in Mountain View, California. Stahl's class features people with varying conditions—acute or chronic pain, asthma, insomnia, cancer, depression, arthritis, stroke. The course includes meditation, gentle yoga, and group discussion. "A lot of things arise—loss, grief, anger, feelings of being overwhelmed. Stress and pain have no age or economic barrier: I'm finding more young people from Silicon Valley in my groups, very stressed out. They sit next to a person who may have minimum mobility or who has had heart surgery. The result is pretty remarkable. Once an individual develops a strong dose of self-awareness, he or she never returns to that place of unawareness. Everyone leaves the course with an ability to cope, no matter their condition."

mates that you require some time alone to meditate. While this sounds easy, for the individual who has never shut the door and asked to have twenty minutes undisturbed, the request can create questions. If questions arise, explain a little bit about meditation and what you are doing. When meditating at home, try to meditate at the same time each day.

Time and Meditation

The best time to meditate is when it is quiet and you will not be interrupted. You can meditate in the morning, afternoon, or evening. Some people meditate in the late afternoon and find that twenty minutes of meditation revives them for the evening. Others prefer to meditate before going to bed, and many meditate in the early morning. The most auspicious times of day to meditate, according to numerous texts on meditation, are at dawn, when the day is fresh and inactive, and at dusk, when all the activity in the atmosphere has settled down.

How Long Should I Meditate?

Don't expect to succeed at settling the mind into a meditative state in a few sessions. Cultivating an effective meditation practice requires time and patience. The longer you spend preparing the mind by studying different methods, defining your goals,

How to Tell If Meditation Is Really Working

• Your mind will feel elevated.

• You will feel more peaceful.

• You will focus better.

• Your quality of life will feel as if it has been enhanced.

• Meditation will be reflected in your actions, thoughts, and attitudes.

and determining what is the right method of meditation for you, the sooner you will be able to sit down and meditate.

The time frame you allot for meditation will depend on your lifestyle. Aim for twenty minutes, but if you can sit for only five or ten minutes, then that is the best place to begin. Don't force your mind to do something it is not prepared to do; it will only grow more restless. If you can meditate twenty minutes, that's a stellar beginning. Perhaps you want to attempt thirty minutes, forty-five minutes, or an hour a day, if you have the desire and the time. It is recommended that you meditate a little each day. It's highly unlikely you will transform the mind into a placid place meditating just once a week. Some words of wisdom from *The Sivananda Companion to Yoga*: "Meditation, like sleep, cannot be taught—it comes by itself, in its own time."

Fitting Meditation into Your Life

Meditation takes discipline. It won't happen without it and it will take time even with it. Once you establish the discipline, and experience the benefits of meditation, it becomes habitual, like brushing your teeth—you do it without thinking about it.

Nevertheless, even the most devout meditator experiences life changes that can interrupt a pretty solid regimen. Something as joyous as the birth of a baby can put a crimp in daily routines. If you find that taking twenty minutes to meditate puts stress on your life at the moment, curtail the time you spend sitting in meditation. The twenty minutes

STREET SMARTS

Sara Myers-Wade began practicing Transcendental Meditation in 1976 and practiced until 1986 when her first child was born. "I thought about meditation, and had every intention of weaving it into my schedule. Then I had a second child. Unfortunately, with two boys and a full-time job, I don't meditate anymore. When I did meditate, I felt my quality of life was much richer. The most I can manage at the moment is to reflect meditatively on the landscape between Bainbridge Island and Seattle when I take the ferry to work five mornings a week."

WHAT MATTERS, WHAT DOESN'T

What Matters

• That you find the best meditation style for you.

• That you are consistent with your practice.

• That you meditate undisturbed.

• That you realize that meditation requires discipline and perseverance.

What Doesn't

• Experimenting with every kind of meditation under the sun.

• That you switch styles or practice a few different styles.

• Explaining meditation to others.

• That emotions come up during your practice.

• That life changes alter your practice.

you had to meditate before the baby was born may have disappeared. In fact, you may feel that the entire day disappears without a moment to rest. Don't berate yourself or feel guilty because your friends with children still manage to meditate. When you are ready to put small increments of meditation back into your life, you will. It may be a walking meditation with your infant, or a reflective meditation in a garden or park. It may happen when you are breastfeeding or closing your eyes for a few minutes in a warm bathtub or doing a breathing exercise. It could take a few months or a few years before you get back to a formal sitting practice.

Meditation and Emotions

When you begin to truly pay attention and concentrate the mind, you may be surprised how little time the mind actually lives in the present. Our emotions romance the mind into the past or future. We agilely identify with our emotions and where they take us. In meditation, the aim is not to engage the mind in the emotions, or thoughts, but to be an unattached witness. When we detach from our thoughts, actions, and emotions without judgment or ego, we recognize that they still exist but they no longer control us. In meditation, the mind acknowledges emotions without entrapment or judgment.

The Result: Life Awareness and Clarity

Meditation involves becoming more aware and more sensitive to what is within you. Regardless of what you experience during meditation, you should be aware of it. Failure to experience peace of mind, mental clarity, bliss, or other ideas you might have about meditation is not a sign that you can't concentrate or meditate properly. What you experience is not important; what is important in meditation is that you are regular with it and that you make an effort. Remain with the object of concentration during your practice, even if your mind wanders. When you see it meandering, gently bring your concentration back to the object.

You need not use any of the above options to meditate. You may be more inclined to find a quiet place, a comfortable position, close your eyes, and relax. Others find walking in nature or viewing a sunrise or sunset a peaceful form of meditation. Whatever meditation technique you choose, remember that it will require some patience, practice, and perseverance. In the end, meditation is what it does for you, not for someone else.

As you can see, both yoga and meditation are highly personal practices. In today's world, yoga is increasingly becoming less gender-specific, as you will see in the following chapters on yoga for women and for men.

THE BOTTOM LINE

Meditation is not about a particular feeling, and there is no one way to meditate, but there are several different techniques. Meditation requires perseverance and patience regardless of which technique you choose. People practice Transcendental Meditation, mindfulness meditation, chanting, gazing at objects, and simple breathing techniques. No longer thought of as New Age quackery, today meditation techniques are incorporated into the programs of numerous health institutions because of meditation's healthful, life-enriching benefits.

....

Yoga for Women

Women practice yoga for a myriad of reasons. Some women discover yoga during pregnancy; others ease into yoga because of menstrual discomfort or for physical as well as spiritual comfort during menopause. There are women who have turned to yoga during traumatic life changes and regard it in a healing light. But the majority of women who do yoga, no matter what their age, practice yoga for personal health or enjoyment. Yoga is the perfect catalyst for harmonizing their body, mind, and spirit.

Yoga and Pregnancy

Congratulations! You're going to be a mom. If you already practice yoga, you may wonder if you should give up your yoga class until after your baby is born. Perhaps you've never done yoga, and pregnancy appears to be the perfect opportunity to begin a class.

According to Elizabeth Bassemir, a prenatal yoga instructor in San Francisco, California, "many women take their first yoga class when they are pregnant. About 75 percent of my students are first-time moms. They want to be around other women experiencing pregnancy."

Pregnancy is a time of joy. It's a journey of miraculous mental and physical changes. Fatigue and nausea may dominate the first few months of pregnancy. Your body begins to change, and so does your attitude about health. While the main goal of prenatal yoga is to prepare for the actual childbirth, practicing yoga during pregnancy can help relieve any discomfort that is associated with pregnancy. Prenatal yoga helps release physical tension in the joints, muscles, and back. By stretching the muscles used in birth, it inherently makes birth easier. In conjunction with the poses, there is plenty of concentration on the breathing practices in preparation for labor.

Prenatal Yoga's Benefits

The benefits of prenatal yoga far outweigh the occasional risk. Many yoga studios and yoga centers have added prenatal yoga classes. Some HMOs and insurance carriers are now offering or covering prenatal yoga classes. The benefits of prenatal yoga are numerous. Cumulatively, prenatal yoga:

• Helps you focus on your pregnancy and your unborn child. Practicing prenatal yoga helps you to discover your inner power and strength.

• Balances the body. Setting aside some time each day to practice breathing exercises and asana nourishes and replenishes the body. This is especially important if you are working or have a busy schedule.

• Improves circulation. In pregnancy, the oxygen-carrying capacity of your blood increases. Your own organs need more blood and the baby and placenta will need approximately one quarter of the blood circulating in your body. This accounts for the breathlessness women sometimes experience during pregnancy. Practicing yoga aids your circulatory system as it does its job.

A Testimonial from Your Author . . .

I had practiced yoga for many years prior to signing up for a prenatal class. My doctor considered my pregnancy to be high risk because I was forty-two years old and a first-time mom. I did not agree with her assessment. Nevertheless, to everyone's surprise, I went into labor six weeks prior to my due date, and sixty miles from my home. I went into the emergency room, where doctors offered concern along with drugs and monitors. Perhaps it was the years of yoga or the prenatal class, but I felt very calm and sure my child would be fine. I said, "No, thank you" and began practicing deep yoga breathing and visualization. The back pains were excruciating, and although the yoga breathing didn't mitigate that pain, it focused my attention away from it. Sixteen hours later I gave birth, naturally, to a healthy little girl. As exhausting as the labor was, I walked out of the delivery room energized.

• Improves breathing. Yoga encourages your breath to flow naturally and normally. It increases energy and vitality. Learning to concentrate on your breath prepares you for difficult moments in labor.

• Helps stabilize emotions. Pregnancy has a dramatic effect on your emotions. You experience incredible emotional transformations. Yoga helps get you in touch with your emotions as well as with the changes in your body.

• Physically prepares the body for the approaching birth. There are certain exercises in prenatal yoga that help the pelvic muscles in preparation for birth. Giving birth is work; yoga helps stretch and prepare you mentally and physically for this very hard, but rewarding job.

When to Begin Prenatal Yoga

As with any exercise program, if you've never done yoga it's best to consult your physician or nurse practitioner. Your body is in constant flux during the first three months of pregnancy. The recommended time to begin a prenatal program is after you have completed the first trimester of your pregnancy, or in your fourth month. Research shows that prenatal problems frequently occur within the first three months of a pregnancy. To err on the side of caution, wait until the beginning of your second trimester to begin a yoga class. Prenatal yoga is different than a regular day-to-day yoga routine.

Consult your doctor before embarking on a prenatal yoga practice, particularly if you are considered high risk or have any health problems.

FIRST: Consult Your Doctor!

It's true, most doctors don't practice yoga, and probably know little about prenatal yoga. Their medical specialty is fetal development and your prenatal health as your body advances in pregnancy. Some women are at higher risk for prenatal problems. Those preparing for multiple births or women who have extremely high blood pressure should always consult with a physician before embarking on a prenatal yoga practice. If your doctor has no knowledge of yoga, ask your prenatal yoga instructor if she can supply you with photos or images of the asana to share with your physician.

Note: Be sure to consult your doctor before you exercise or practice prenatal yoga if you have any of the following factors:

- Hypertension

- Toxemia

- Diabetes

- Risk for premature labor

Prenatal Yoga Practices to Do

Prenatal yoga helps relieve stress and prepares the body and the mind for the birth process. In a typical prenatal class you will practice the following:

- Standing postures

- Sitting or kneeling postures

- Pelvic floor exercises

- Restorative poses

- Breathing

- Visualization and meditation

Prenatal Postures to Avoid

There are certain postures that you should avoid during pregnancy. You might read or come across photos that show women in what looks to be precarious postures for the pregnant body, such as a head stand, or shoulder stand. Many of the women in these photos are yoga instructors or have practiced yoga for many years. They may modify the postures, or they feel confident enough with their bodies to practice such poses. However, it is not recommended that pregnant women practice the following types of poses.

- Do not practice inverted postures, or poses that turn the body upside down.

A Note to the Reader:

The types of postures and poses (and some of the specific poses) mentioned in this chapter are found earlier, in chapter 4, "The Asana," pages 55–104.

• Avoid poses that stimulate the abdomen a great deal. Likewise, avoid poses where you must lie on your stomach.

• Avoid intense twisting poses.

• Avoid supine poses after the twentieth week.

• Avoid jumping into poses.

• At the first sign of bleeding or cramping, discontinue yoga (or any exercise, for that matter) and call your doctor.

• Come out of any pose that feels stressful.

Inverted Poses to Avoid

While inverted poses have many health benefits, it is best to avoid them during pregnancy. They reverse the blood flow in your body. You should not come across inverted poses in a prenatal class. If you already practice yoga, it's best to discontinue these poses or asana during pregnancy. The inverted poses are:

• The Head Stand (Shirshasana)

• The Shoulder Stand (Sarvangasana)

• The Plow (Halasana)

• Bending forward where the crown touches the floor.

Abdominal Poses and Breathing Exercises to Avoid

You will not be able to do poses on your abdomen. Your instructor may alter some of the poses or use props. When stretching, do so with care. Avoid extreme stretching positions which may pull on the abdominal area. Pregnancy is a wonderful time to stretch the body, but not strenuously.

Breathing exercises should be gentle and gradual in prenatal yoga. Avoid the rapid or intense breathing exercises, such as:

• Kapalabhati

• Bhastrika

Supine Poses to Avoid

After the twentieth week of pregnancy it is not advisable to do supine poses. Positioned between the abdomen and back are major vessels that carry blood. Lying on your back can impede this flow of blood and so reduce oxygen delivery to the placenta.

Pregnancy also puts stress on your lower back. The enlarged uterus stretches the abdominal muscles so that they can no longer support the lumbar spine. As your pregnancy advances, your center of gravity changes and is pulled forward. This forward pull strains the lumbar spine or lower back. Postural awareness helps this and so does practicing squatting exercises.

Relaxation Poses to Avoid

During your second trimester of pregnancy you will have to forgo the Savasana (Corpse Pose; Relaxation pose). There are other options for this wonderfully relaxing pose that your instructor will teach you. One is a modified Corpse Pose where you rest on your side with pillows for support. The other is a restorative pose with blankets, bolsters, and pillows.

Don't assume that what felt easy to do and relaxed in your twentieth week of pregnancy will feel easy and relaxed in your thirtieth week. As your body grows, so will your repertoire of prenatal poses and your prenatal ingenuity.

Pregnancy, Gravity, and Yoga

Your center of gravity shifts during your pregnancy, and so does your center of balance. In preparation for childbirth, the body releases a hormone called relaxin that aids in the delivery process. Relaxin allows the ligaments and tendons to stretch more easily. However, the release of relaxin also reduces the muscular and ligament support in the body, increasing the likelihood of strain during exercise.

In Your Final Weeks of Pregnancy

As the birth of your baby approaches, your body begins to feel heavy. The pressure of the growing baby pushes on your organs. They feel scrunched together, making it difficult to sleep. As the baby moves into the birth position its head may push on a ligament called the round bone, causing irritation. The magic of pregnancy often turns to fatigue a few weeks before your baby's birth. Your body is sending you an important message—relax and rest whenever you can. You may want to shorten your yoga practice, or do simple restorative poses.

Menses and Yoga

Women experience extraordinary cycles throughout their lifetimes. Because of hormonal patterns, menses, childbirth, and menopause, a woman's life is an intricate passage of magical cycles. Nevertheless, women don't always ease through the cyclical galaxy without emotional or physical interruption. The first awakening of a woman's cycle begins when she is a young girl with menstruation, often before she ever comes across the word "yoga."

Every month, until the onset of menopause or during pregnancy, a woman ovulates, releasing eggs in preparation for pregnancy. When pregnancy does not occur, a self-cleansing process, called menstruation, occurs. Some women breeze through menses with little or no discomfort. But many experience mental and physical discomfort caused by the fluctuation of hormones or stress. This discomfort is known as premenstrual syndrome or PMS. Women experience PMS in varying degrees, but some of the more common symptoms associated with PMS are the following:

- Bloating

- Back pain

- Irritability

- Depression

- Breast tenderness

- Food cravings

These are unpleasant passages for the women experiencing these symptoms. Having a regular yoga practice helps relieve many of these symptoms, or curtails the intensity of them.

Yoga provides immediate relief for discomfort and an opportunity for inner renewal. Some of the asana help relieve physical discomfort from cramps and back pain, while others ease emotional tension. Because the body is naturally cleansing or moving matter out, avoid inverted poses during menstruation.

Helpful Asana for PMS

The following exercises are helpful for PMS:

- The Cobra (Bhujangasana)

- The Cat (Bidalasana)

- The Relaxation Pose (Savasana)

Perimenopause and Menopause

Within the next twenty years, upwards of 40 million American women will enter menopause. Menopause can occur between the ages of thirty-five and sixty. The approximate age of menopause hovers around the ages of fifty to fifty-five. Prior to menopause, women experience perimenopause. This is not the same as menopause; it is premenstrual tension from delayed menses. In perimenopause, the

STREET SMARTS

Mood shifts are not a new phenomenon to Ariela Wilcox. "I've battled PMS forever, but when perimenopause started, I felt like Attila the Hun—my friends ran for cover. I began eating differently and exercising, but it wasn't until I added meditative practices from yoga that I really felt balanced and in control. I chant and meditate daily. It's an integral part of my life."

menstrual cycle is erratic. The shifting levels of estrogen and progesterone, both mood-altering hormones, frequently result in a host of uncomfortable emotional and physical changes. Perimenopause, like menopause, can trigger:

• Anxiety

• Manic mood swings

• Muscle aches and joint aches

• Stiffness

• Erratic sleep patterns

Menopause is the secession of a woman's menstrual cycle, the end of her reproductive cycle. Some common complaints of menopause are:

• Vaginal dryness

• Hot flashes

• Urinary problems

• Mood swings

• Depression

• Fatigue

• Disturbances in sleep patterns

Researchers have begun to recognize that ancient disciplines, such as yoga and meditation, are valuable assets during these passages. In our society, many women fear and loathe the onset of menopause. It can become a time of great consternation instead of a meaningful rite of passage. Practicing yoga inspires a spiritual awakening and empowers a woman as it awakens the body to its strength, flexibility, and natural wisdom. Women who have practiced yoga prior to menopause find the onset of both perimenopause and menopause easier or report less discomfort associated with these cycles. Yoga can help combat the emotional and physical stress that is often a part of menopause.

Yoga to Address Anxiety

The stretching in yoga increases joint mobility. The combination of the postures and meditation helps to tone and soothe the sympathetic nervous system and relieve anxiety.

Yoga to Address Hot Flashes

Scientists are not sure what causes hot flashes. Some speculate that the body's temperature goes awry when the hormones fluctuate. Nevertheless, in certain societies, such as Japan, hot flashes are relatively rare. There is no word for "hot flash" in the Japanese language. In America, nearly 80 percent of women report experiencing hot flashes. Inverted poses, which cause the flow of blood to reverse direction, appear to have a measurable effect on the glands of the endocrine system that regulates hormone levels.

F.Y.I.

If you have not practiced inverted postures or have never done yoga, do not try them on your own. Always seek a good teacher. If you have a neck injury, spinal injury, or hypertension, do not practice inverted postures. A knowledgeable teacher can help you with modified inverted postures.

STREET SMARTS

Robin Montgomery
discovered yoga in the
1970s while going
through a divorce. "I
took a class in some-
one's home. We were
six women, a small,
intimate group, and I
loved it. It helped me
get through the
emotional turmoil.
Later I began taking
classes at the Self-
Realization Center in
Encinitas, California.
Although I do not
practice yoga regularly,
the principles are still
very much a part of my
lifestyle—tranquillity,
an ability to not let
stressful situations
derail my life, and a
sense of peace."

Yoga to Address Hormonal Fluctuations

Practicing yoga can help address underlying hormonal changes that produce anxiety and moodiness. Stress, poor nutrition, and hormonal shifts are associated with:

- Low libido

- Fatigue

- Depression

- Mood swings

These tend to deplete the adrenal glands. During menopause the ovaries stop producing progesterone and estrogen; however, estrogen continues to be manufactured by a number of other organs, such as the adrenal glands and kidneys. Practicing yoga poses—such as the Half Spinal Twist, lying on the floor and bringing your knees to your chest, or backward poses such as the Bow Pose—helps to stimulate the kidneys and adrenals.

Yoga to Address Mood Swings and Depression

Mood swings are a common complaint during both perimenopause and menopause. They are uncomfortable and, some women report, uncontrollable.

One way to help alleviate insomnia, irritability,

and depression associated with menopause is to practice soothing postures. Poses with forward bends, such as Uttanasana (see page 62) or Janu-Shirshasana (page 71), soothe the mind and calm the nervous system. These poses stretch the spine and place a gentle, reassuring pressure on the abdomen and uterus.

Yoga to Address Bone Deterioration

One of the consequences of menopause, due to the decrease of estrogen, is osteoporosis. Osteoporosis literally means "porous bones." Lifestyle can play an important role in osteoporosis, but so can certain medications that have a debilitating effect on bones. Weight-bearing exercises and a healthy diet are vital to aging bones, but yoga can also play an important role in both stress management and posture. A woman's frame can actually diminish with osteoporosis. Rounded backs, slumped shoulders, and vertebral fractures often contribute to the collapse of vertebrae. Practicing yoga assists with spinal alignment.

There's no solid, worthwhile reason for women to wait to begin a yoga practice in order to manage moods, stave off bone loss, or assist with any of the other numerous proven benefits that yoga offers women. Yoga, for many people, both women and men, is an injection of inspiration—no matter what passage or cycle of life one may be in or happen to be going through. A yoga class might not kiss PMS good-bye forever or help you conquer

SMART SOURCES

National Osteoporosis Foundation
1150 17th St., N.W. Suite 500
Washington, DC 20036-4603
(800) 223-9994
www.nof.org

America's leading source for women seeking up-to-date, medically sound information on causes, prevention, detection, and treatment of osteoporosis.

perimenopausal anxiety for good, but it will certainly rejuvenate you and inspire the relationships around you.

With all these benefits for women, what about the benefits of yoga for men? Men may not take up yoga to combat brittle bones, PMS, or for fatherhood, but many men do practice yoga for a variety of reasons and find it equally rewarding. Do real men do yoga? Of course; let's look at chapter 8.

THE BOTTOM LINE

Yoga can gracefully assist women through menses, premenstrual syndrome, pregnancy, childbirth, and perimenopause and menopause. Prenatal yoga is different from a daily yoga practice; you should not begin a prenatal class until after your first trimester, and you should not start without the guidance of a prenatal yoga instructor and your doctor. Then you can practice yoga up until delivery. Yoga is a potent practice to nurture the female mind and body through all their changes.

Yoga for Men

With the advent of yoga's popularity and its numerous benefits, more men than ever are taking and teaching yoga, making the exercise even more accessible.

When yoga instructor Roger Eischens, a runner, four-star athlete, and former university football coach, took his first yoga class in 1969 for stretching, a handful of men were interested in yoga. Eischens, who teaches an offshoot of Iyengar yoga called energy yoga says athletes are incredibly strong but lack the flexibility and balance that yoga can give them. "I work from the premise that yoga is the basic movement that prepares one for anything they want to do; yoga makes all things accessible."

Do Real Men Do Yoga?

If you're a typical North American male, you work long hours and experience a fair amount of stress during the day. Nevertheless, you try and balance this stress with a workout, or incorporate fitness into your routine. You feel confident that between work, family, and friends you manage just fine. You're surprised that your annual physical reveals alarmingly high blood pressure. Your doctor suggests some dietary restrictions and pills. But your girlfriend or wife suggests the unthinkable—a yoga class!

But is it all that "unthinkable"? Surprise! It's not, simply because the benefits of yoga are not gender specific. Millions of men the world over regularly practice yoga, and most were attracted to yoga for many of the same reasons:

- Because someone suggested it, or a friend does it and swears by it

- To reduce stress

- For weight loss

- To enhance sports performance

- Out of sheer curiosity

- To search out something more life enriching

- To augment spirituality

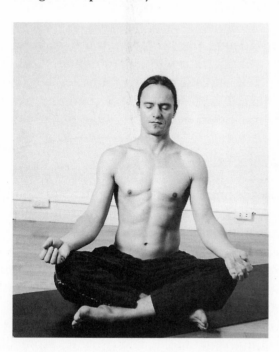

SMART SOURCES

Roger Eischens
Sports Kinesiology,
  Yoga
P.O. Box 4035, Ryan
  Rd.
Blue Mounds, WI
  53715
(608) 767-3931
www.uwmf.org/living/
  library/sports/yoga.
  htm

Looking for information on athletics and yoga? Try contacting Roger Eischens, a yoga instructor and kinesiologist in Blue Mounds, Wisconsin. Roger, an athlete and former football coach, studied Iyengar in India.

STREET SMARTS

After twenty years on the road as a country-western musician, Bill Hendrick left the music industry to work in art restoration. Four years into his new profession, he was diagnosed with chronic fatigue syndrome. "I became obsessed with a spiritual path. I parked myself in metaphysical bookstores and read everything I could. I met an old friend and discovered that our spiritual experiences had some similarities. She was practicing siddha yoga, a very traditional yoga based on a guru-disciple relationship, which incorporates the study of Vedic texts, raja yoga, meditation, chanting, karma yoga, and to a lesser extent hatha yoga. I began reading Mutananda's books, the founder of siddha yoga, and have studied with his disciple who came to the West, Swami Gurumayi, for the last ten years."

Yoga Myths

In India, traditionally men teach yoga, and they are credited with importing yoga to the Western cultures. In America the opposite occurred—it is primarily women who have taught yoga classes, although this is rapidly changing; more men are teaching yoga than ever before. For both men and women who practice yoga the psychological benefits are a given. But physiologically women tend to have more suppleness and balance going into yoga. Men have strength, yet their athletic training has ignored their body's alignment, balance, and suppleness.

The following are some of the more common reasons for men to embark on yoga. Also given are rebuttals to myths about yoga.

- **Yoga is not wimpy.** Au contraire, yoga requires concentration, strength, determination, and stamina. The payoff isn't bigger muscles, but balance and flexibility. A thirty-minute routine can stretch every muscle in your body. Some of the postures require great strength. (See the Peacock Pose, Mayurasana, on page 90.)

Charlie Jones, an airline employee who hurt his back lifting, has been doing the Sun Salutation for six years. "It's all I do in the morning, besides a few push-ups. I had no idea I was doing yoga when I started it, and I don't practice yoga otherwise. I've suffered for years from a bad back, and a friend suggested I try this exercise. He didn't call it the Sun Salutation, but when I purchased a tape to better understand the sequences, I realized I was doing yoga and it had a name. I practice it pretty regularly, but only twice each session, once for each side of my body. If I skip a few days, my back acts up, so I'm pretty disciplined."

• **Yoga is not too hard.** Yoga is like anything else that you begin: the more you do it, the easier it becomes. What can be difficult for men is getting beyond the idea of competition. Yoga is not competitive or about winning. You don't check your pulse, heart rate, or length of practice. Yoga does, however, emphasize precision when doing the poses.

• **Yoga is cerebral as well as physical.** Yoga encourages self-acceptance. No matter what type of yoga you practice, it will encourage integration of the body, the mind, and the soul. There are many different types of yoga. You may find hatha incompatible with your personality, and you might fare better in a raja yoga or bhakti yoga class.

• **Yoga relates to everyone's life.** Even if your first experience with yoga was less than satisfying, the point of yoga is about *your* life. Some men don't relate to the style of some women instructors or a particular yoga philosophy of the teacher. If this has been the major roadblock to yoga for you, seek out a class taught by a man, or take a weekend yoga retreat for men only. Even among male teachers techniques differ.

• **Yoga does not have to be about gurus.** Yoga is sometimes used by devotees as a spiritual practice. Many practices are teacher-guru based. That doesn't mean you have to follow a guru or practice a particular type of yoga. There are many generic yoga classes that are not guru based. Classes taught at the YMCA, health clubs, or gyms are typically not attached to a specific yoga lineage.

STREET SMARTS

"When I began yoga thirty years ago, it did not occur to me that it would be a constant thread throughout my life and work. As an undergraduate student at UC Berkeley, I had experimented with different types of yoga and meditation groups. While I was in medical school at Baylor, in Texas, I read *Autobiography of a Yogi.* I went to classes and practiced kriya yoga when time permitted. During that hectic period of my training, and currently, my yoga practice affords my mind a quiet dwelling, a sense of ultimate relaxation," says James F. Zucherman, M.D., medical director of St. Mary's Spine Center, San Francisco.

A Scenario: "Everyman's" First Yoga Class

You're open-minded and even though the idea of sitting with your legs crossed or hoisting yourself into a position with your feet in the air is not appealing, you go to a yoga class. The first impression is not a good one. Too many lithe bodies, and mostly women, in the class, all effortlessly rolling forward to touch their heads to their knees. Their hands fall in line and appear comfortably glued to the ground. They are graceful doves making the movement look simple. It's not simple, and the three men in the class struggle to inch their arms toward the top of their kneecaps. The instructor mumbles something about breathing into the pose and relaxing. Everyone is breathing and stretching. Not you; you're sweating and stiff. Thankfully, the class closes with something called yoga nidra, or deep relaxation—the entire class collapses on their backs like a corpse. After class, the woman next to you informs you that you snored through the entire deep relaxation. Wasn't that the purpose? you ask. Nix yoga!

Unfortunately, this type of scenario is too often a man's first encounter with yoga. The lesson to be learned is simple: Don't despair. As any yogi will tell you, it will take time. And the old sports adage rings true here as well: Practice makes perfect.

• **Regular guys do yoga too.** Given the misconceptions that many have about yoga, it isn't surprising that you might be skeptical. But real men do practice yoga and meditation, including athletes, coaches, rock singers, and doctors.

• **The analogy of hatha shouldn't make you nervous.** Just talking about uniting energies and the balancing of the feminine and masculine contained in oneself may be a new concept to the linear way of thinking. While the outcome of a yoga practice is the numerous physical and mental benefits discussed throughout this book, yoga also allows the outer rejuvenation to affect your inner core. It's a window, if you want to open it, to your inner landscape.

• **Sleep and stress reduction do not do the same things for you as meditation and deep relaxation.** Sleep is very nice and necessary, but it has nothing to do with stress reduction or yoga. Practicing yoga or meditation has been documented to improve circulation, respiration, digestion, the cardiac system and blood pressure, and a constellation of other positive benefits.

• **Yoga is not a sport.** Yoga is not a sport; it should never be practiced as such. Yoga will, however, stretch and lengthen muscles and loosen your joints.

If you're an athlete, yoga may seem strange for several reasons—there is no team, no winner and loser, no shaking hands or patting on the back. Being noncompetitive is not easy for men to accept—it goes against the grain of the entire social structure for many men, from sports to the workplace. You may have been told that if you don't compete you won't get ahead. Yoga is not about getting ahead. Instead, it deposits fertile seeds for growing a healthy body and mind and inner personal development, whether you work on Wall Street or take care of the kids at home.

Many good athletes lack flexibility and range of motion in their bodies. Lifting weights, for example, does not require flexibility, nor does tossing the ball around in the front yard with your kids. As the body ages, so does its mechanisms—the shoulders may slump from too much time sitting, the spine loses its freedom of movement, and leg muscles tighten up. Yoga helps the tendons, muscles, and ligaments to retain elasticity. Another benefit

WHAT MATTERS, WHAT DOESN'T

What Matters
• That men can attain a sense of well-being from yoga.

• That you try different types of yoga classes to experience what style best suits you.

• That yoga, like a sport, requires practice and perseverance.

• That you give yourself permission and time to practice yoga if you want to.

What Doesn't
• Being flexible or able to touch your toes.

• Being athletic.

• Already playing a sport—yoga is not a sport. nor does it preclude your playing of sports.

• That most men you know don't participate in yoga or show the least bit of interest.

• That your first yoga class was a snore.

of yoga often overlooked, yet clearly a part of professional athletic training, is concentration and the value of focusing the mind.

Men, like women, incorporate yoga into their lifestyles for a variety of reasons, such as a general sense of well-being, calmness, and increased strength and endurance. Emotionally, men find yoga to be a marvelous conduit for bridging blocked or dormant emotions. With more medical institutions delving into how the emotions interact with the body and mind, men who have stoically borne the burden of stress and heart disease are some of the first to understand the benefits of yoga.

If your doctor suggests that you practice yoga or meditation, if you are under tremendous stress, or you have back pain or concerns about your health, turn the page.

THE BOTTOM LINE

Men approach yoga for different reasons. It may be at the suggestion of a doctor or spouse, or because they are interested in physical flexibility. Some men find that yoga enriches their inner lives, and for some it guides them through life transitions. If your first experience with yoga was not a positive one, try another class or another style of yoga. Men sometimes resonate with some of the more physical styles of yoga.

Yoga and Health Concerns

In the last decade yoga has become a part of clinics and hospitals to help manage a variety of chronic diseases and disorders, both physical and mental. Yoga is now the foundation for several stress reduction programs around the country.

Yoga and Mainstream Medicine

Good health is the fruit of a yoga practice, so it is no surprise that the health benefits from hatha yoga and meditation have been successfully incorporated to treat or augment some clinical conditions, from heart disease to the relief of chronic pain. While yoga has long been a part of Ayurvedic medicine, it is only just beginning to make inroads to Western medical institutions. Where skepticism and doubt have been put aside by traditional Western clinicians, the results have made headlines.

The Cost of Stress

Stress is linked to hypertension, heart attacks, diabetes, asthma, chronic pain, allergies, headaches, and insomnia. The costs to industry from dealing with stress-related ailments has hit the $200 billion mark, and even individuals who are not ill find that stress dominates their lives. Debbie Hamolsky, an oncology nurse in San Francisco, was prompted to explore yoga during a collaborative work effort with Dean Ornish's program. "My schedule is so hectic that, although I had been meaning to take yoga for years, something always came up. I opted for this weeklong retreat, and grumbled about what I needed to do as I drove to the retreat. Indeed, I was stressed when I arrived, but after a week of relaxation, a lot of yoga, meditation, and an enormous amount of time sitting still, I felt my body and head relax in an extraordinary way. It was a 110 percent positive experience. I still don't have time for a yoga class, but I manage to practice relaxation from tapes."

What Yoga Can Offer the Afflicted

Yoga's multifaceted approach to life and health offers restorative energy, hope, strength, and inspiration in times of illness and for those afflicted with an injury, migraines, repetitive strains, or a life-threatening condition.

Life begins with the breath, and breath, of course, is what sustains life. As Alice Hodge, author of *Taking Charge of Your Health,* points out, yoga is about connecting our inner core with our breath:

"Practicing yoga is what makes me feel the best at this time," says Hodge, who was diagnosed with a rare form of cancer and has undergone eight surgeries in less than a decade. "I practiced yoga before I was diagnosed with cancer, but it has become a vital part of my life. Yoga has been an immense support emotionally for both my family and me. I go to classes when I can, and at home I rely on the restorative poses to help me sleep. The

F.Y.I.

40 million Americans have cardiovascular disease.

60 million Americans have high blood pressure.

80 million Americans have elevated levels of cholesterol.

For one-third of the population, the first indication that they have heart disease is a heart attack.

Source: Dr. Dean Ornish's Program for Reversing Heart Disease

breathing practices and imagery have guided me through some difficult moments; they've also given me strength and a very positive outlook on my life."

Yoga and Heart Disease

No one in the field of cardiology took yoga to heart twenty years ago. It was an accepted article of faith among cardiologists that coronary heart disease was progressive and irreversible: the conventional wisdom was that if you had coronary heart disease, it would only get worse. This gloomy prediction for poor health troubled Dean Ornish, a resident at Baylor Medical School in Texas. One evening at his parents' home in Houston he was introduced to a man by the name of Swami Satchidananda. Doctor Ornish began studying yoga with Swami Satchidananda, whom he credits with triggering his pioneering work in the reversal of heart disease. Ornish's program includes a very-low-fat diet, yoga, meditation, relaxation, and exercise.

A maverick in the field of reversing heart disease, the Ornish program is now in hospitals around the country, and the book *Dr. Dean Ornish's Program for Reversing Heart Disease* is used by countless patients. Many of Dr. Ornish's patients who commit to his program are initially reticent and scared, much the way Werner Hebenstreit, one of the original subjects in Dr. Ornish's first pilot study, was thirteen years ago.

Yoga's Proven Benefits in Helping Those with Coronary Heart Disease

When Werner Hebenstreit met Dr. Ornish, the seventy-one-year-old had suffered two heart attacks, four failed angioplasties, and had an intense disdain for doctors. When Dr. Ornish called and asked Werner to consider being part of the original experimental program on heart disease, Werner said he wasn't interested.

"I was a miserable old man, an invalid. I had always been active physically and mentally. Now I couldn't walk across the street without chest pains. When Dr. Ornish said, 'You really have nothing to lose, Werner, give me a four-week commitment to the program,' I entered the program."

Werner walked through the door of the Preventive Medicine Research Institute in Sausalito, California, a complete skeptic. "Yoga was not new to me, I had lived in India decades ago. I had no interest in yoga or meditation, but I wasn't a stranger to those sciences," recalls Werner.

Dr. Ornish's program is a drastic departure from other heart disease ideologies. It required Werner and the thirteen other heart patients to practice elementary yoga postures, relaxation, and meditation, along with strict dietary changes and mandatory group discussions at the end of each session. Spouses were encouraged to attend the program.

"The first time the yoga instructor told me to lie on my back, I was sure I would never get up again. In retrospect, the hardest part of the program wasn't the yoga or meditation, but talking about feelings. I realized that I didn't know a

STREET SMARTS

International yoga instructor Amy Gage, former coordinator of Lifestyle Heart Trial Research for the Dean Ornish Preventive Medicine Research Institute, says: "I feel basically that we are spiritual beings, once we can scratch the surface, which happens in yoga. Particularly if one has a life-threatening disease, it allows people to get in touch with their inner lives. Teaching yoga has always been a transforming experience for me as an individual and as a yoga teacher."

SMART SOURCES

Preventive Medicine
  Research Institute
900 Bridgeway
Sausalito, CA 94965
(415) 332-2525

thought from a feeling. To sit and grapple with feelings in a group was much more difficult than stretching my body forward or calming my mind. It took a lot of prying to open my heart. Today, my wife and I travel all over the world lecturing for the Ornish program. I guess you would say I'm an Ornish convert. I even speak on national television, and when the yoga teacher can't teach our weekly yoga class, I'm the instructor. Life, at eighty-four, has never been better or healthier."

Yoga and Chronic Pain

Around the same time Dean Ornish was in Texas pursuing his theory on the reversal of heart disease, Massachusetts scientist Jon Kabat-Zinn, Ph.D., had a zany notion of introducing the principles of yoga and mindful meditation into a stress clinic for chronic pain. In 1994 his success was featured on the PBS Bill Moyers special "Healing and the Mind." Today, 250 hospitals around the country have implemented Jon Kabat-Zinn's mindfulness program.

Kabat-Zinn, who is executive director of the Center for Mindfulness in Medicine at the Stress Reduction Clinic at the University of Massachusetts Medical Center, has an approach to chronic pain that emphasizes gentle yoga and mindfulness meditation. The success of the program relies on a process. The process isn't always easy; the requirement is not that one like the process but that one simply does it.

For eight weeks, people afflicted with varying

Integrative Yoga Therapy (IYT)

Integrative yoga therapy combines various yoga traditions with an emphasis on yogic therapeutic approaches and techniques for health-related fields. While an in-depth understanding of yoga postures is essential for working with individuals, a thorough knowledge of mind-body health science is mandatory. Many of the country's most knowledgeable yoga teachers, some of whom are mentioned in this book, are members of Integrative Yoga Therapy and participate in workshops and programs for those interested in pursuing the IYT teacher training program. Several IYT instructors hold advanced degrees in physical therapy, psychology, or health education.

Integrative Yoga Therapy offers training programs with an emphasis on applying yoga to the needs of individuals and groups with specific medical problems. The courses include teaching methodology and mind-body health sciences. For information, contact:

Joseph Le Page, M.A.,
Executive Director of Integrative Yoga Therapy
Integrative Yoga Therapy
P.O. Box 238
Blue Lake, CA 95525
(800) 750-9642

degrees of chronic pain, from crippling pain to psychological stress, are carefully guided through a sequence of gentle hatha yoga, breathing practices, and mindful meditation. The class encourages a moment-to-moment awareness. The yoga postures emphasize nonstriving. The program works to cultivate the wisdom to self-liberate from pain and suffering, a very different concept for a culture that instantly wants to anesthetize pain.

SMART SOURCES

Stress Reduction Clinic
University of Massa-
    chusetts Memorial
    Health Center
55 Lake Avenue N.
Worcester, MA 01604
(508) 856-2656

Mind/Body Medicine
    Clinic
2440 E. 5th St.
Tyler, TX 75701
(903) 592-2202

Awareness and Relax-
    ation Training
Santa Cruz Medical
    Clinic
2025 Soquel Ave.
Santa Cruz, CA 95062
(408) 458-5530

Stress Management
    Clinic
The Chopra Center for
    Well-Being
7630 Fay Avenue
La Jolla, CA 92037
(888) 424.6772
Emphasis on the body-
mind-spirit connection

Association of Trans-
    personal Psychology
P.O. Box 4437
Stanford, CA 94305
(650) 327-2066

Yoga and Back Pain

Back pain results from a variety of complex factors, from congenital disorders to poor posture to injury. The condition of your spine affects your entire body. Many people suffer from severe back ailments caused by stress. Stress depletes the oxygen in your body. When the muscles cannot get enough oxygen to nourishes them, they spasm. The way we sit, stand, and move all can create potential problems for our spines.

Both the breathing practices and the asana increase the oxygen in our bodies. Practicing asana stretches the spine and keeps it supple. But if you already suffer from a bad back, or have had back surgery, you may fear hurting your back in a yoga class. Nor is the idea of sitting in a meditation pose appealing if you have a bad back. For spinal problems it is paramount that you find a class specifically designed with your back in mind. This is not to say that your average yoga instructor does not have a working knowledge of the back, but postures and asana need to be altered for back problems.

Back Problems? Issues and Questions to Consider Before Taking Up Yoga

Between your neck and buttocks lies a huge chunk of anatomical landscape. And if you have back problems, it's best to talk with a yoga teacher before you embark on a class. Explain as specifically as you can your back dilemma and any concerns you may have. Ultimately, ask what experience the teacher has had in teaching students with back pain. Here are some other issues to explore with your instructor:

• Do you have a cervical, thoracic, or lumbar problem?

• Have you had surgery or do you have fused vertebrae?

• Does your spinal injury stem from an accident?

• How fearful are you of movement?

• Do you have acute or chronic back pain or a severe genetic problem?

• How will you master meditation practices or breathing practices if you cannot sit for long periods of time?

• Are there pillows and blankets available to support your back?

Yoga and Carpal Tunnel Syndrome

If you work on computers, play an instrument professionally, or do any type of repetitive movement, you are at risk for carpal tunnel syndrome. Carpal tunnel syndrome occurs when the median or mid-

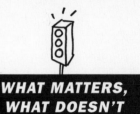

WHAT MATTERS, WHAT DOESN'T

What Matters
• That you approach yoga as a treatment to medical problems with an open mind.

• Being willing to integrate yoga into your traditional health modalities.

• Yoga may not cure chronic pain, but it may ease it.

• That you find a yoga teacher who has experience teaching individuals with your condition.

What Doesn't
• Your history of success or failure with other treatment modalities.

• That you're a little skeptical.

• Your age.

• That your insurance carrier doesn't acknowledge yoga.

dle nerves, which are in an enclosed compartment bound by the carpal bones, are compressed. Increased pressure within the tunnel from repetitive movement aggravates the syndrome. Carpal tunnel occurs more commonly in women than men, probably due to the fact that women have smaller carpal bones and less tunnel space than men.

A February 1999 study published in *The Lancet* medical journal examined eleven yoga postures for the arm, each held for a specified amount of time, along with relaxation. After eight weeks, the grip strength was significantly better and pain reduction greater in those who did yoga than in those who didn't. One of the primary positions was the Namaste, or Prayer Position.

Namaste
(Prayer Position)

Here's a simple exercise to do to help ward off the damaging effects of carpal tunnel syndrome. If you have carpal tunnel syndrome or arthritis in your wrists, keep the forearms together during this exercise.

1. Bring the hands in front of the chest, gently joining the palms and fingers together. Your forearms should not be touching and your elbows are slightly extended.

2. Firmly press the palms together and hold for 2 counts, then relax.

3. Again press the palms together and spread the fingers against each other and firmly press together. Hold for the count of 2, then bring the fingers back together and relax.

Yoga and Arthritis

Yoga will not cure arthritis, but it will help restore joint flexibility and strengthen movement. Practicing yoga will help prevent the degeneration of healthy joints.

Yoga and Health Insurance

As evidence of the health benefits of yoga continues to mount, some insurance carriers and HMOs are beginning to cover yoga. At Kaiser Permanente, one of the largest HMOs serving the United States, yoga and mindful meditation classes are offered through the Health Education Services Department. Nancy Bouffard, director of Kaiser Permanente's health education services in San Francisco, says the classes do not concentrate on or adhere to one style of yoga, but demonstrate a variety of yoga postures with an emphasis on stretching, toning muscles, relieving tension, and cultivating mind-body awareness. Not all Kaiser Permanente sites around the country offer yoga, but a growing number do. Although the classes are not free, the fee is nominal for members and only a bit more for nonmembers.

While this chapter explored some of yoga's contributions to the health field, the last chapter of the book shows yoga's full spectrum—it takes yoga into the workplace, on the road, and from the wide-eyed wonder of a child's vision of yoga to the amazement and beauty of seniors practicing yoga.

THE BOTTOM LINE

Yoga is very good medicine, and it doesn't require a prescription. It is a good antidote for chronic pain, back pain, arthritis, and even some life-threatening illnesses. Many clinics and hospitals recognize yoga's healing abilities for individuals, and classes are cropping up in health care facilities across the country, some of which are subsidized by insurance coverage. Many yoga teachers become yoga therapists, specializing in one or more forms of healing yoga. People with illnesses or chronic pain should investigate the potential yoga may have in helping them deal with their conditions.

Yoga: The Peripatetic Practice

Reading and learning about yoga is easy. The essence of yoga is balance, humming along without watches or worry. It takes a modicum of creativity and commitment to find that balance. The truth is that it is a challenge to eke out a corner of our lives for yoga with our chaotic schedules. Between marriage, the kids, baseball practices, swimming lessons, relocation, and business trips, the full calamity of living doesn't offer much time to toss a sticky mat on the floor and melt into the Corpse Pose.

Yoga will not turn calamity into pleasure, but it is a catalyst for change and peace of mind. Threads of yoga can weave surprising results into an arduous day. If you truly want to practice yoga, start with where you are at this moment. You may have to sprinkle a dash of ingenuity into the yoga menu. Let's start with those of you who are always on the road.

Yoga for the Traveler

On the road again? Nothing interrupts a routine more than travel, unless it's for pleasure. It's one thing to go to St. Lucia to snorkel and soak up some rays and quite another to go to St. Louis for a meeting. Admittedly, when you are sprawled under a palm tree sipping piña coladas, yoga may not be necessary. But if you're one of the millions who flies for business and spends an inordinate amount of your day sandwiched in an airplane seat or stranded in a passenger terminal, threading yoga into your itinerary can ease travel tension.

Yoga helps the body adjust to the rigors of

travel, both physically and emotionally. Start basic, with your breath. The Three-Part Breathing technique (see page 43) can be done anywhere. You may not have any control over delayed flights or crowded planes, but you do have some say over your breath.

And any chance you get to move around and stretch your legs during a flight will help your circulation.

So now you're sitting on the runway, shoulder-to-shoulder with two strangers, stuck in the middle seat. You question if it is viable to practice yoga in such a tiny space. After all, you're accustomed to doing yoga in a cozy studio with people you know or at home with soft lights and silence.

Yoga makes all things possible. Wherever you are, begin by centering yourself with your breath. Put your feet flat on the floor and your hands on your lap. Close your eyes. Let's do some airport asana.

The Grounding Breath

This simple breathing exercise is a technique many savvy travelers who don't like to fly use for take-off.

1. Center your attention.

2. Close your eyes and concentrate on your breathing. Begin by exhaling. Inhale, allowing the breath to rise from your belly and fill the chest cavity before the air rises into your lungs. Exhale, taking longer than you did with the inhalation.

3. If you use a mantra, repeat it silently.

The Seated Stretch

This stretch, good for your back and neck, is a variation on the Seated Chair Stretch illustrated on page 69.

1. Your spine should be erect and stomach muscles tucked in.

2. Stretch your arms straight over your head,

SMART SOURCES

A good way to ease the stress of travel is to pack a cassette player in your carry-on and purchase a guided relaxation tape. Music stores and bookstores carry some of these cassettes. If you would like to order through a catalog, Living Arts has a wide selection of tapes, videos, and music available.

Living Arts
P.O. Box 2939
Dept. YJ502
Venice, CA 90291
(800) 582-6872
  (24-hour fax)
www.livingarts.com

palms facing each other. Interlace your fingers, except for the index fingers.

3. The index fingers, which are touching, stretch upward, giving the spine a good stretch. Do not lift your shoulders or roll your head back.

4. This stretch elongates the spine. Don't forget to breathe.

Seated Twist

This easy practice, a variation on the Chair Spinal Twist illustrated on page 87, opens the upper body.

1. Space permitting, move slightly forward in your seat.

2. Bring your hands behind your back and clasp your right wrist with the left hand, and the left wrist with the right hand. If you cannot reach your wrists, clasp your hands.

3. Inch your hands toward your elbows, opening the chest. Breathe.

Eye Yoga

Eye movement exercises are perfect for airplanes and offices.

1. Begin by looking straight ahead. Move your eyes up and down without moving your head. Practice a set of twelve.

2. Then keeping your head straight, move your eyes side to side. Do not move your head. Practice a set of twelve, then relax the eyes.

3. Finish the sequence by looking straight ahead and moving your eyes clockwise in a circle. Imagine that your eyes are acknowledging each number on the face of a clock. Repeat the move counterclockwise. Practice these moves six times in each direction. When you are finished, rub your palms together briskly as you would on a chilly day. Cup the palms over your eyelids and relax. Hold for sixty seconds and breathe. Eye yoga relaxes the eyes and energizes the mind.

Standing Half-Spinal Twist

This pose can be done in an airport while you wait for your luggage or at your hotel.

1. Stand straight, put your left hand in the small of your back, and extend your right hand upward, palm turned toward your head.

2. Feet together, gently twist the body, taking the head and shoulders to the right. The lower half of your trunk remains straight. Do not push, but gently stretch. Return to center and repeat for the opposite side.

Remember: No matter what city you are in, there will always be a yoga studio or yoga classes. This is an opportune time to drop in and discover a new class. If you travel to a particular destination a great deal, search for a yoga class that you can drop in on on an irregular basis.

Yoga in the Workplace

Okay, you've reached a milestone, you can sit in a half lotus pose, touch your toes, and you can meditate for longer than fifteen minutes. Nevertheless, the lack of time in your schedule is beginning to cramp your yoga style. Your new job requires more business trips than usual and you're at the office more than you are at home. When will you find time to practice yoga? The solution to your time crunch is the workplace.

According to yoga instructor Dee Benefield, who has taught yoga for nearly fifteen years, "More and more corporations are adding yoga classes at the demand of their employees. The workplace has become very stressful. Many corporations have a gym on site in which yoga classes are taught. Employers are looking for ways to mitigate workplace stress, and more and more employees are looking for a yoga class. Most of the classes I teach are at lunch or after work. There is a tremendous demand for yoga in the workplace."

The evidence that yoga boosts morale and productivity on the job is mounting. People in the workplace gravitate to yoga because they are stressed, and yoga makes them feel better and helps them manage stress. Clarity and creative thinking are boosted, and in the long run, so is overall job effectiveness.

If your company does not offer on-site yoga, pull up a chair and take a five-minute break. Do this five times during the course of the day and you have incorporated twenty-five minutes of yoga into your day. The following exercises are powerful stretches to relieve computer-related tension. The poses alleviate tension in the neck, back, arms, and upper body.

Seated Chair Stretch

(This office stretch is illustrated in chapter 4, on page 69.)

1. Sit on the edge of a chair in your office. Make sure the chair does not swivel.

2. Put your left hand behind your back, the palm turned away from your back. Stretch the right arm upward.

3. Take the upward extended hand and reach behind your back to grasp the left hand. Hold and breathe into the stretch.

4. Repeat for the opposite side.

Note: One side of your body will probably be more flexible than the other side. The stretch is difficult and you may not be able to reach the other hand. Stretch only as far as you can. Use a handkerchief or a towel in the upward stretched arm and allow the hand behind your back to grasp it. This will aid the stretch.

Chair Spinal Twist

(This office stretch is illustrated in chapter 4, on page 87.)

1. Sit on the edge of your chair. Your spine should be erect.

2. Reach around with your left arm and place it on the back of the chair or behind you.

3. With your right arm, reach across the front of your body and twist, turning the upper torso to the left. Breathe and release.

4. Repeat for the opposite side.

Neck Stretch

1. Sitting erect in a chair, look forward.

2. Gently stretch your neck to the right side.

3. Leading ever so gently with the left arm, stretch that arm down the left side of the body. Breathe into the pose and hold for ten or fifteen seconds.

4. Repeat for the opposite side. This stretch gives the neck and shoulders a nice stretch. Try this pose at home, sitting on the floor in the Easy Pose. Sitting on the ground allows a more extended stretch.

Standing Stretch

1. Stand straight in Tadasana, facing the wall.

2. Bend your right leg at the knee, toes toward the buttocks. Reach around with your right hand and grasp the right foot or ankle with the right hand. Balance with your left hand against the wall if you need support. Stretch for a count of fifteen to thirty seconds.

3. Breathe into the pose, and release. Repeat for the opposite side.

Yoga for Children

You must be kidding! Your child never stops moving. She makes a bumblebee look lethargic. Well, that's what children do, they move around, and if you allow them, they will teach you just how creative yoga can be.

Marsha Wenig, creator of the *YogaKids* video and educational curriculum, says that when you are teaching kids yoga, you have to instill in them that they have roots and wings. "It's important to grab their attention. You can't teach yoga to children the same way you teach yoga to adults; it is too boring for their active minds, they want none of it. They expect a lot of creativity, little talk and a great deal of action. An instructor has to be very present and sensitive. You have to lead kids into the movement with things they can relate to. For example, when I teach the snake posture or cobra, I have the kids draw it, then tell me how it feels to be a snake. Before we do the pose, I ask them to show me how a

SMART SOURCES

If you are interested in seeing how creative yoga can be for children, the *YogaKids* video, the winner of the Parents' Choice award, is entertaining and informative for children. If you would like more information on the *Yoga-Kids* video or the YogaKids certification program, contact Marsha Wenig at:

Dancing Feet Yoga
   Center
2501 Oriole Trail
Long Beach IN 46360
(219) 872-9611
(800) 968-0694

Another yoga video for little ones is *Yoga for Children*. For a catalog or video, contact:

Shakticom
Rt. 1, Box 1720
Buckingham, VA 23921
(800) 476-1347

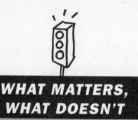

WHAT MATTERS, WHAT DOESN'T

What Matters
• That children don't always remember what you taught them on a given day, but they do remember who taught them and how you taught them.

• Giving children simple directions.

• That you give gentle reminders and not harsh criticism.

• Remaining mindful that they *are* children and are most likely not interested in adult-style yoga.

What Doesn't
• That children have a lot of energy or are eager to show you how to do yoga.

• That children do yoga with regularity.

Source: YogaKids Facilitator Certification Program 1997 ©

snake climbs a tree without any hands, and then imagine what the snake must be thinking. After that, they can't wait to do the pose."

Ageless Yoga

A whopping number of the population is galloping toward fifty. This segment of our society, the baby boomers, will live longer than any generation before them and consider themselves the fittest generation on the planet. Nevertheless, many move into midlife with stress-related ailments and a host of physical problems once reserved for those decades older.

Yoga is not a cure for any disease, nor is it a magic bullet for ailments, but in conjunction with proper health habits you couldn't ask for a better companion to age with. Lilias Folan, author of *Lilias, Yoga, and Your Life,* wrote that "yoga is for everyone, at any age. You can begin at any time of your life. If you are over sixty-five, there is no better time to start."

Practicing yoga, many seniors discover the miracle of their bodies for the first time. Others are fascinated at just how good they feel, and for many, yoga is a natural extension of an already healthy lifestyle. Yoga is ageless.

Some Tips for Older Yoga Newcomers

If you are a senior and new at yoga or taking your first yoga class, here are some suggestions:

- Seek out a class in which a majority of people are around your age. Seek out a teacher who has experience with teaching seniors.

- Begin with a gentle style unless you are athletic.

- If you have any health problems or concerns, speak with your doctor before embarking on a yoga class.

- If you have high blood pressure, avoid inverted poses.

- If you have osteoporosis, be careful of placing stress on brittle bones.

- If you have arthritis, you may need to move at a slow, gentle pace.

SMART MOVE

Indra Devi is one of the century's most renowned yoga teachers. Indra was born in 1890 and was the first foreign woman to study yoga with masters in India. During an interview in her nineties she was asked, "How does it feel—aging?" Devi replied, "I don't know how it feels. Ask someone who's aging. I don't know anything about aging."

Source: The New Yoga for People Over 50, Suza Francina

Yoga Retreats

Something magical happens at a yoga retreat. Suddenly you find yourself amidst like-minded strangers, people that have come together to practice yoga. The atmosphere is calm, conducive to reflection and relaxation. You practice yoga a few times a day, meditate, hike, and relax. A retreat is a wonderful way to regenerate and savor your energy; it's also the perfect place for deepening a yoga practice. For many individuals a retreat is a restful repose from life; for others it is a life-changing experience.

There are hundreds of yoga retreats in both hemispheres to rejuvenate mind, body, and spirit. The settings are often spectacular. Retreats vary in price. They can range from $35 to $3,500, and

The Mindful Body

Ten years ago, Roy Bergmann was an avid runner and a successful commercial banker. He also suffered with terrible back pain. He recalls those years as some of the most stressful in his life. "My days revolved around deadlines. The chiropractor I was seeing for back pain suggested yoga. Athletic, I opted for a more strenuous yoga style, which turned out to be fine. I practiced yoga religiously and became interested in health. Over time, I felt calmer inside, but outside my life was in unforeseen turmoil. I went through a divorce. My company merged and my job disappeared. I had the resources to stop and reflect on my life. Instead of looking for another job, I decided to follow what I really wanted to do—create a business that incorporated yoga and health, a sanctuary where people could feel comfortable. Five years ago I opened The Mindful Body in San Francisco, California. It is not a health club, but it offers many different levels and styles of yoga classes, body work, meditation, and a place for workshops. I even added a small spa for people to use."

For more information on The Mindful Body, contact:

Roy N. Bergmann
The Mindful Body
2876 California St.
San Francisco, CA 94115
(415) 931-2639
www.themindfulbody.com

from a humble, simple retreat site to exotic surroundings. There are yoga retreats in the Yucatán and Alaska, in Bali and Hawaii, and in your own backyard. You don't have to go exotic to reap the benefits that a retreat offers, so look locally.

Some of the retreats are expensive; many more are reasonably priced. Some offer a specific style of yoga or meditation; others offer a variety of practices and styles. Retreats often feature a special yoga instructor or instructors that come to facilitate or teach special workshops. Here are some types of retreats that you might consider.

Day Retreats

A day retreat lasts an entire day. Most are silent retreats (see below). Lunch may be included or you may be asked to bring a vegetarian bag lunch. A day retreat can be at a yoga center, an ashram, or in a stunning country setting.

Silent Retreats

Not all retreats are silent. A silent retreat, however, is just that—you don't talk during the day. Silence allows the mind to relax and to pay attention to what is happening inside of you.

Short Retreats

Before you cash in your annuities to travel halfway around the world for a retreat, it may be more sensible to first try a short retreat closer to home. Many ashrams and yoga studios offer short retreats. This is also a good introduction to the idea of retreats.

One- or Two-Week Retreats

These are longer retreats and a little more intense, time-wise and cost-wise.

Month-Long Retreats

Many ashrams offer longer retreats, and teachers' training programs are typically a month or longer. Some of the ashrams offer family-style retreats, others do not.

F.Y.I.

Do you live near a resort or health spa or do you frequent health spas? If so, you may want to ask about yoga classes. Many luxury resorts, such as Meadow Wood in Napa Valley, offer yoga classes for their guests in the spa. Not surprisingly, local residents in the valley discovered the yoga class, which encourages local participation.

SMART SOURCES

Set on thirty-five acres
in northern California,
the Yoga Research
Center is the first of its
kind in the country. Its
founder, Georg Feuer-
stein, is one of the
foremost yoga scholars
and the author of
numerous texts on
yoga. For more infor-
mation, contact:

Yoga Research and
   Education Center
P.O. Box 1386
Lower Lake, CA 95457
(707) 928-9898
www.yogaresearch-
   center.org

What Are You Paying For?

Day retreats are the most economical. The price of
any retreat is often dictated by what the retreat site
offers. When looking for a retreat, here are some
cost-conscious things to ask:

• **Location.** Is it on an island, in front of the
ocean, in the mountains, close to home, or does it
require extensive travel?

• **Accommodations and food.** Are the rooms private or do you share quarters? How many people
are in a room if you share? Are the meals basic or
gourmet? Do you prepare your own meals or is
food included in the retreat package?

• **Can you camp?** This can cut down on cost.

• **What's included?** Do you need to bring anything special?

• **Yoga style.** Will the retreat focus on one style of
yoga? Is it compatible with what you want to do?

• **What level is it?** Is it a retreat for beginners or
for advanced students and teachers? Are the yoga
levels mixed?

• **Who'll be teaching?** Is the retreat offering
workshops or yoga classes with a well-known yoga
instructor?

Yoga in Health Clubs

Yoga instructor Suzanne Deason from Rolling Hills Health Club in Novato, California, has been practicing yoga for thirty-five years. You may have seen Suzanne on yoga videos or remember her from Richard Hittleman's yoga program on television. Currently, Suzanne, along with several other distinguished yoga instructors, is working on a protocol or type of certification for yoga teachers. "In health clubs, I find that many of my students are athletic and come to class with injuries. Others approach yoga as they would a sport. They are very flexible and want to maximize every pose. I explain to them that yoga will make you flexible, but yoga is not just about flexibility. One student who could do a perfect Bound Eagle with his knees on the floor asked me how he could maximize the pose. I said, 'What are you ever going to do in your life that requires you to use your knees in that way?' I think it is important to bring the spirit of yoga, its benefits, and kinesiology into health clubs. It's important to hire trained teachers who have a background in yoga and kinesiology. Not everyone who teaches yoga in a health club is a yoga teacher; standards vary."

Spas and Wellness Centers

The 1990s have seen a proliferation of wellness centers and spas around the world. A wellness center integrates a holistic path to wellness and offers various programs, from yoga to stress reduction. The medical personnel are usually trained in mind-body medicine, and doctors on staff address health concerns.

A visit to a spa might replenish the mind, body, and spirit, but a spa is not a medicinal setting. People frequent a spa in this country for pleasure. European spas have a medicinal component that is often covered by their insurance system. While some spas in North America are pampering palaces, others focus more on health. Yoga has become popular in spa programs around the world. Optional yoga classes are part of both spa resorts and day spas. If you live near a spa, you may be able to participate in yoga classes given there.

Yoga in the New Millennium

Despite the long-standing and steadily growing public interest in yoga, there are few organizations in the West or East dedicated to the objective study of yoga and the various aspects of its traditions. In 1996, Georg Feuerstein, renowned yoga expert, established the Yoga Research Center. The center is dedicated to preserving the traditional teachings of yoga, promoting research, and maintaining a library. The center offers degree programs and teacher training programs and collaborates with other yoga research and education centers around the world.

If you were to ask a yoga master what yoga is, he or she would talk of yoga's essential nature and its profound wisdom, spiritual integrity, and effective healing powers. If posing the same question to a child who practiced yoga, the child would most likely describe yoga in graphic, succinct terms—a mighty mountain, a candle, or a tiny seashell. A senior might venture to say that yoga is a beloved companion or the fountain of youth. The individual who suffers with chronic pain might express yoga as a getaway to great joy. For numerous individuals, yoga cannot be expressed verbally; it is enough to say that it feels like a vast, fenceless landscape of inner peace and joy.

THE BOTTOM LINE

Even if you have a hectic lifestyle, with a little ingenuity you can practice yoga anywhere, no matter who you are. There are asana suitable for airplanes and airports, for children and for seniors. Ultimately, you may want to deepen your yoga practice or learn more about yoga by attending a retreat. There are hundreds of retreats and many superb yoga teachers around the world. If you don't want to wander too far away from home, you may prefer to retreat to a nearby spa or health club and check out what it has to offer in the way of yoga.

Index

Body:
awareness of, 8, 10
balance of mind and. *See*
Mind/body connection
getting in touch with, 57
heat in, 131
limb for control of, 13
mind distinct from, in
Western medicine, 127
Bolsters, 123
Bone deterioration, 156, 169
Botanical practice, for
focusing the mind, 144
Bouffard, Nancy, 189
Bound Eagle Pose (Baddha
Konasana; Butterfly Pose),
67
Bow Pose (Dhanurasana), 76,
168
Brain, 30, 81, 133
Breathing:
awareness of, 58
back pain and, 186, 187
cycle of, 42, 43
deep, asana for, 79
exhalation in, 35, 42, 43,
44, 47, 141
ineffective, 40-41
inhalation in, 35, 43, 47
mental state and, 41, 53
stress and, 40, 41
TM's affect on, 145
walking and, 143, 144
see also Pranayama
Breathing Book, The (Farhi),
48
Breathing exercises, 47-53
Bhastrika (Bellows Breath),
52-53, 162
Full-Breath, 48-49
Grounding Breath, 193
Kapalabhati (Skull Shining
Breath), 51, 162
Nadi Sodhana (Alternate-
Nostril Breathing
Exercise), 50-51
Single Nostril, 49
Warming up the Breath, 48
Bridge Pose (Setu Band-
hasana),
78
Buddhism, 148

Business sector. *See*
Workplace, yoga in
Butterfly (Baddha Konasana;
Bound Eagle Pose), 67

Calm mind, 2
asana for, 66, 68
Cancer, 181-82
Cardiovascular disease, 148,
181
see also Heart disease
Cardiovascular system, 8, 9,
177
breathing and, 41
Carpal tunnel syndrome, 180,
187
Prayer Position (Namaste)
and, 187
Cassettes, relaxation, 194
Cat Pose (Bidalasana), 94, 165
Center for Training in
Mind/Body Medicine, 127
Certification, for yoga
teachers, 110, 111, 124,
205
Chair Spinal Twist
(Bharadvajasana), 87, 198
Chakras, 126-36
in astral body, 126, 129
blocked, 129
clearing, 134-36
continual movement within,
126
described, 126
prana absorbed and
distributed through, 126,
129, 131, 136
seven major points, 128-34
twenty-one minor points,
129
Western vs. Eastern
philosophy and, 126-28
yoga without working with,
134
Chanting, 14
in kundalini yoga, 30
in meditation, 46-47, 153
in Sivananda yoga, 31
Chest:
asana for, 75, 79
breathing and, 43, 44
Chi, 39

Children, yoga for, 192,
199-200
resources for, 199
Child's Pose (Mudhasana), 92
Cholesterol level, 181
Chopra Center for Well-Being,
186
Choudhury, Bikram, 26
Chronic pain, 2, 3, 8, 108,
180, 184-85, 188
Circadian rhythms, 126
Circulation, 8, 177
asana for, 81, 84
breathing and, 41
chakras and, 131
prenatal yoga and, 157
Clarity, meditation and, 139,
153
Classes. *See* Yoga classes
Clothing, 57, 112
Cobra (Bhujangasana), 77, 165
Colors, chakras associated
with, 133
Commercialism, 121-22
Communication, chakra of, 132
Comparing oneself to others,
114
Compassion, 132
Competitiveness, 175, 177
Complementary and Alternative
Medicine Program, Stanford
School of Medicine
(CAMPS), 148
*Complete Illustrated Book of
Yoga, The* (Devananda), 30
Concentration, 22, 60, 138
asana for, 66, 84, 88, 90
athletic performance and,
178
chakras and, 132
meditation techniques
focusing on, 140, 147-48
sensory input and, 140
Confusion, 133
Consciousness, center of,
133-34
Coordination, 57, 60
Coronary Heart Disease
(CHD), 8, 9
inverted poses and, 81
yoga's benefits for, 180,
182-84

Books in the
Smart Guide™ series

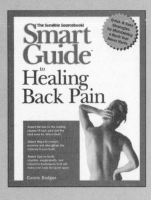
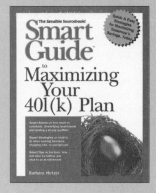
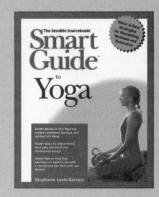
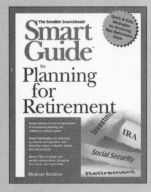
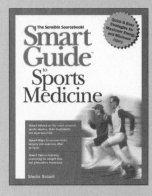
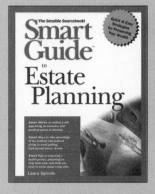

Smart Guide™ to
Estate Planning

Smart Guide™ to
Healing Back Pain

Smart Guide™ to
Maximizing Your
401(k) Plan

Smart Guide™ to
Planning for Retirement

Smart Guide™ to
Sports Medicine

Smart Guide™ to
Yoga

Smart Guide™ to
Boosting Your Energy

Smart Guide™ to
Buying a Home

Smart Guide™ to
Getting Strong and Fit

Smart Guide™ to
Getting Thin and
Healthy

Smart Guide™ to
Healing Foods

Smart Guide™ to
Making Wise
Investments

Smart Guide™ to
Managing Personal
Finance

Smart Guide™ to
Managing Your Time

Smart Guide™ to
Profiting from Mutual
Funds

Smart Guide™ to
Relieving Stress

Smart Guide™ to
Starting a Small Business

Smart Guide™ to
Vitamins and Healing
Supplements